AF710817

GEISINGER

Geisinger Clinic is a multispecialty physician group practice with nearly 650 physicians located in central and northeastern Pennsylvania. The clinic's mission is "to enhance the quality of life through an integrated health service organization based on a balanced program of patient care, education, research, and community service." This mission is summarized: **"Heal. Teach. Discover. Serve."**

To learn more about the Geisinger Healthcare System visit www.geisinger.org

*FAQs** SERIES

Also in this series

Current Titles

Low Back Pain FAQs

Rheumatoid Arthritis FAQs

Weight Management: Childhood and Adolescence FAQs

Weight Management: Adults FAQs

Menopause FAQs

Upcoming Titles

Asthma FAQs

Hypertension FAQs

Headache FAQs

Insomnia FAQs

Diabetes FAQs

---

*Frequently Asked Questions

DEPRESSION

GEISINGER

FAQs

Authors
Susan L. Paolucci, MD
Stephen J. Paolucci, MD

Series Editor
Sandra A. Buckley

2007
BC Decker Inc
Hamilton

BC Decker Inc
P.O. Box 620, L.C.D. 1
Hamilton, Ontario L8N 3K7
Tel: 905-522-7017; 800-568-7281
Fax: 905-522-7839; 888-311-4987
E-mail: info@bcdecker.com
www.bcdecker.com

07 08 09/PI/9 8 7 6 5 4 3 2 1

ISBN 1-55009-370-3
Printed in Canada

Sales and Distribution

United States
BC Decker Inc
P.O. Box 785
Lewiston, NY 14092-0785
Tel: 905-522-7017; 800-568-7281
Fax: 905-522-7839; 888-311-4987
E-mail: info@bcdecker.com
www.bcdecker.com

Canada
BC Decker Inc
50 King Street East
P.O. Box 620, LCD 1
Hamilton, Ontario L8N 3K7
Tel: 905-522-7017; 800-568-7281
Fax: 905-522-7839; 888-311-4987
E-mail: info@bcdecker.com
www.bcdecker.com

Foreign Rights
John Scott & Company
International Publishers' Agency
P.O. Box 878
Kimberton, PA 19442
Tel: 610-827-1640
Fax: 610-827-1671
E-mail: jsco@voicenet.com

Japan
Igaku-Shoin Ltd.
Foreign Publications Department
3-24-17 Hongo
Bunkyo-ku, Tokyo, Japan 113-8719
Tel: 3 3817 5680
Fax: 3 3815 6776
E-mail: fd@igaku-shoin.co.jp

UK, Europe, Scandinavia, Middle East
Elsevier Science
Customer Service Department
Foots Cray High Street
Sidcup, Kent
DA14 5HP, UK
Tel: 44 (0) 208 308 5760
Fax: 44 (0) 181 308 5702
E-mail: cservice@harcourt.com

Singapore, Malaysia, Thailand, Philippines, Indonesia, Vietnam, Pacific Rim, Korea
Elsevier Science Asia
583 Orchard Road
#09/01, Forum
Singapore 238884
Tel: 65-737-3593
Fax: 65-753-2145

Australia, New Zealand
Elsevier Science Australia
Customer Service Department
STM Division
Locked Bag 16
St. Peters, New South Wales, 2044
Australia
Tel: 61 02 9517-8999
Fax: 61 02 9517-2249
E-mail: stmp@harcourt.com.au
www.harcourt.com.au

Mexico and Central America
ETM SA de CV
Calle de Tula 59
Colonia Condesa
06140 Mexico DF, Mexico
Tel: 52-5-5553-6657
Fax: 52-5-5211-8468
E-mail: editoresdetextosmex@prodigy.net.mx

Brazil
Tecmedd Importadora E Distribuidora De Livros Ltda.
Avenida Maurílio Biagi, 2850
City Ribeirão, Ribeirão Preto – SP – Brasil
CEP: 14021-000
Tel: 0800 992236
Fax: (16) 3993-9000
E-mail: tecmedd@tecmedd.com.br

India, Bangladesh, Pakistan, Sri Lanka
Elsevier Health Sciences Division
Customer Service Department
17A/1, Main Ring Road
Lajpat Nagar IV
New Delhi – 110024, India
Tel: 91 11 2644 7160-64
Fax: 91 11 2644 7156
E-mail: esindia@vsnl.net

Notice: The authors and publisher have made every effort to ensure that the patient care recommended herein, including choice of drugs and drug dosages, is in accord with the accepted standard and practice at the time of publication. However, since research and regulation constantly change clinical standards, the reader is urged to check the product information sheet included in the package of each drug, which includes recommended doses, warnings, and contraindications. This is particularly important with new or infrequently used drugs. Any treatment regimen, particularly one involving medication, involves inherent risk that must be weighed on a case-by-case basis against the benefits anticipated. The reader is cautioned that the purpose of this book is to inform and enlighten; the information contained herein is not intended as, and should not be employed as, a substitute for individual diagnosis and treatment.

Introduction

Depression is more than just the "blues." It's a serious, debilitating illness that can cause profound suffering—even death. It affects millions of Americans, and takes a grave toll both on those who have it as well as their families. Depression also costs the economy millions of dollars a year in lost productivity and disability.

Most people still don't understand that depression isn't a personal weakness or a character flaw but a medical illness that can be treated and controlled, leading people back to wellness. Without proper treatment, depression can last for months or even years. It can lead to other medical conditions or make existing conditions worse. Ultimately, some people commit suicide to escape their pain, unleashing further pain and suffering on their families and friends.

Depression is an *illness*-not a *weakness*. People shouldn't be ashamed to admit they are ill. Depression is *treatable*—and patients *can* feel well again—all the way well.

About This Book

This book can help people understand what depression is—and what it isn't. After reading this book, people should understand:

- The symptoms of depression
- What causes depression
- Who depression affects, including the special populations of children, women, and the elderly
- Different treatments for depression
- Suicidal thinking and behavior
- Concrete suggestions for the families and loved ones of depressed patients to help them get well
- How to use available resources and references for further information

This book isn't intended as a substitute for careful evaluation and treatment by a health care provider. It's intended as a place to start to understand this common, terrible, but treatable illness.

At the end is a glossary of terms related to depression.

Contents

CHAPTER ONE

What Is Depression?

Depression is more than just the "blahs" or the "blues." It's a persistent feeling of sadness that doesn't go away. It's like a dark cloud that settles into your brain despite everything you have tried to get rid of it.

What are the symptoms of depression?

Q

A

Nearly every episode of depression has certain symptoms that last at least 2 weeks, including:

- Extremely low moods
- Sadness
- Loss of interest or pleasure and
- Severe problems functioning at home or at work, or with relating to others

Depression may include other symptoms, too (Table 1-1). We list even more symptoms of depression in Chapter 2 when we start to talk about the different types of depression.

No matter which symptoms a person is having, the bottom line seems to be that those who are depressed feel hopeless or empty inside. Reassurance doesn't seem to convince them that they might get better. Some may even spend the entire day in bed, or not be able to sleep at all.

Are the symptoms of depression all emotional?

Q

A

No. As you can see in Table 1-2, many sufferers will have physical symptoms (like headaches, upset stomach, or chronic pain) that don't seem to respond to usual treatment. Not every person will experience every symptom and symptoms may vary in how severe they are and how long they last.

Table 1-1: Defining Depression

These symptoms are almost always present, and last at least 2 weeks to be considered depression:

- Extremely low moods
- Sadness
- Loss of interest or pleasure and
- Severe problems functioning at home or at work, or with relating to others

Other common symptoms:

- Problems sleeping or eating
- Low energy
- Problems thinking clearly or concentrating
- Feeling either slowed down or anxious
- Feeling overly guilty or worthless or
- Having recurrent thoughts of death or suicide

Table 1-2: Depression: More Than Mental

- Physical symptoms that don't seem to respond to treatment
- Common ailments are headaches, upset stomach, chronic pain
- Not everyone with depression will have the same physical symptoms and some will have no physical symptoms at all

Q

Is depression common?

A

Yes. Depression is one of the most common illnesses in the country, and can affect up to 12% of men and 25% of women at least once in their lifetime. In the United States, 19 million people are diagnosed with depression every year. Family physicians will see that 15 to 25% of their patients have some degree of depression at any given time. More people in the United States have depression than have heart disease, cancer, and AIDS combined! Despite this, more dollars in this country are spent per person per year on tooth decay ($11), heart disease ($130), and muscular dystrophy ($1,000), than depression ($10) (Fig. 1-1).

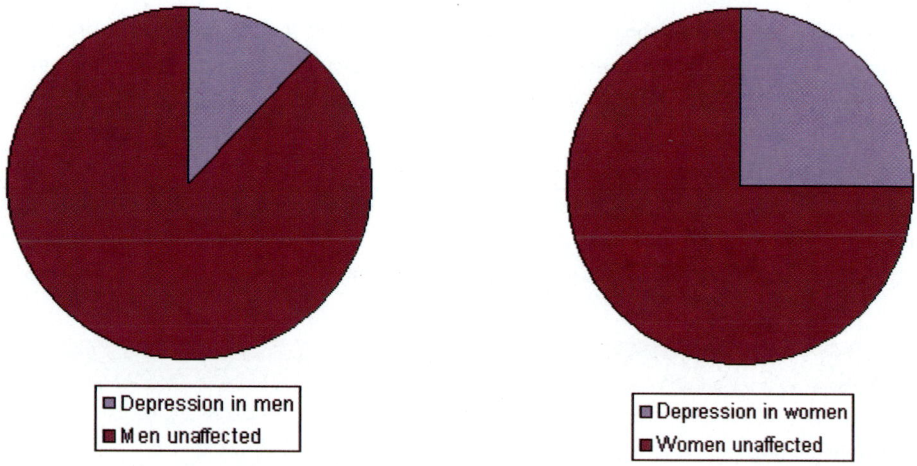

Figure 1-1. Depression rates in the United States: up to 12% of men and 25% of women.

Does something "trigger" depression?

Depression might be triggered by a life stress or a loss, but it can also settle in when things are going well. This is the danger of depression—people don't seek help because they think that they "shouldn't" feel this way, that others have it worse, and that they should be able to pull themselves up and get out of this on their own.

In Good Times and in Bad

Depression might be triggered by a life stress or a loss, but it can also settle in when life seems perfect and things are going well.

Can a person "snap out of" depression?

No. That's like saying that someone with cancer can just pull themselves out of their disease! Depression, like cancer, is a medical illness that is treatable. Depression, like cancer, isn't a personal weakness or a character flaw. It has a usual set of symptoms that lasts for weeks and causes major problems in how a person functions. Without treatment, these symptoms can last for weeks, months, or even years. Without treatment, depression can even be fatal.

Is psychosis the same thing as depression?

No. Some people suffer from *psychosis*, which means being out of touch with reality. They may hear voices that aren't really there or feel paranoid or suspicious. They may suffer from *delusions*, which are false beliefs that can't be shaken: "My body is putrid and rotting." "I am so evil that the government is coming to get me and kill me." Reasoning with them doesn't change their thinking, and as their suffering intensifies, they may withdraw in fear from those who are trying to help them. People who are psychotic or suicidal represent true psychiatric emergencies and need immediate evaluation and care to keep them safe and save their lives.

Do most people with depression seek help?

Studies show that over half the people suffering from depression are never diagnosed or treated! Sadly, the longer someone suffers, the harder it is to get them all the way well.

Like most diseases, does depression have an economic impact?

Yes. Because of depression, millions of dollars are wasted every year from workforce and productivity losses. Currently, depression ranks second only to heart disease in terms of its economic impact on society, and it's soon expected to be number one. From the human perspective, we can't calculate the cost of suffering. Over 30,000 depressed people kill themselves every year, including over 2,000 children and adolescents. We'll discuss this more in Chapter 8.

Is this why it's so important to diagnose depression and get people into treatment?

Yes. Like a ripple in a pond, depression touches not just the sufferer but those who care for him or her. People die from this illness, not just by their own hand, but because depression can worsen other physical illnesses like heart disease or cancer. With early detection and treatment, lives can be saved and terrible burdens lightened.

Q

A

Haven't some well-known people suffered from depression?

Yes. We can learn much from people who have courageously come forward with public accounts of their struggles with depression. Think of folks like Terry Bradshaw, former quarterback for the Pittsburgh Steelers and four-time Super Bowl winner. Bradshaw battled his own war with the stigma of depression for years, thinking that successful professional athletes "shouldn't" be depressed. There's also Barbara Bush, former First Lady, who spoke explicitly about her fight with suicidal thoughts, and her shame that a woman with a "perfect" life such as hers could be depressed.

Words of Comfort From Those Who Have Been There

Sufferers can take comfort from the words of William Styron, the award-winning author who wrote about his own struggles with depression:

"To most of those who have experienced it, the horror of depression is so overwhelming as to be quite beyond expression...if depression had no termination, then suicide would, indeed, be the only remedy. But...depression is not the soul's annihilation; men and women who have recovered from the disease—and they are countless—bear witness to what is probably its only saving grace: it is conquerable."

—Styron, William. Darkness Visible: A Memoir of Madness.
New York: Random House, 1990

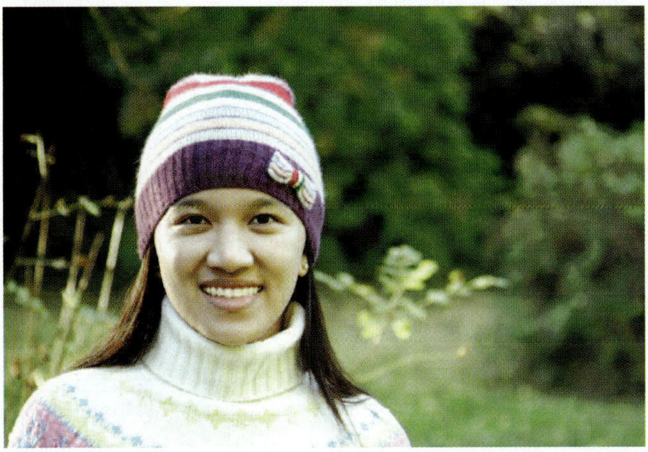

all the way well

CHAPTER TWO

What are the Different Types of Depression?

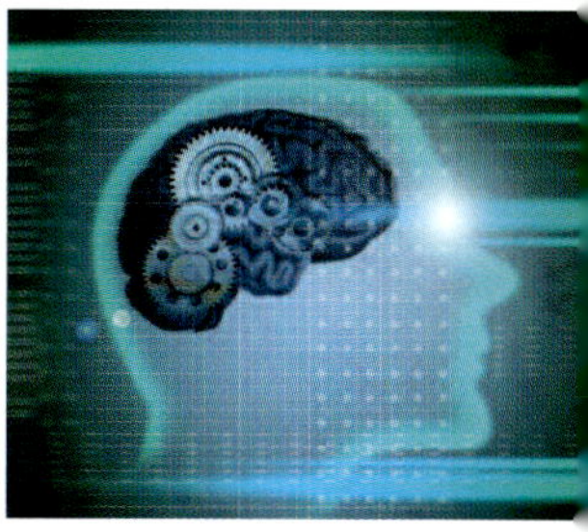

Just as there are many types of cancer or arthritis, there are different types of depression too. It's important to know what type of depression one has because this plays an important role in determining what kind of treatment is best. Milder types of depression might respond to counseling alone or exercise and lifestyle change alone. More severe types of depression might need both medication and counseling, or even other forms of therapy.

Depression Isn't "One Size Fits All"
Just as there are many types of cancer or arthritis, there are different types of depression.

What are the different types of depression?

Q A

Depression is classified as:

- Major (also known as clinical or unipolar)
- Minor (dysthymia)
- Bipolar disorder

Each has a recognized set of symptoms.

What is major depression?

Q A

Major depression (sometimes called *clinical* or *unipolar* depression) includes a recognized set of symptoms (Table 2-1). Major depression can be diagnosed if a person is disabled by sadness and five of the other recognized symptoms for at least 2 weeks. Someone who is depressed doesn't have to have all of these symptoms, but the symptoms they do have will last for weeks, not days, and severely interfere with their ability to live well and function. Some people may have one episode of major depression, but most have several in their lifetime, especially if they aren't treated.

Can major depression lead to psychosis?

Q A

Serious depressions can have psychotic symptoms such as:

- Severely disorganized thinking
- Appearing to be irrational and incoherent

Table 2-1: Symptoms of Depression

- Feeling sad, empty, nervous for a long time
- Feeling hopeless, helpless, pessimistic
- Problems sleeping, waking early in the morning and unable to get back to sleep
- Loss of interest or enjoyment in hobbies, activities previously enjoyed
- Feeling worthless, guilty, overwhelmed, inadequate
- Feeling tired, lazy, no energy or zest
- Problems concentrating, thinking clearly, remembering things
- Ambivalence, can't make decisions
- No appetite with weight loss or overeating with weight gain
- Agitation, irritability, physical restlessness
- Loss of interest or enjoyment in sex
- Persistent thoughts of death or suicide
- Physical symptoms (such as headaches, stomach distress, chest pain, chronic pain) that won't go away despite treatment

- Speaking but not making sense
- Experiencing *auditory hallucinations* (voices telling them they are bad)
- Having *delusions* (false, unshakable beliefs that mirror a person's low self-esteem and hopelessness)

Some examples of delusions might be:

- A feeling of "rotting inside," corresponding to feelings of guilt and worthlessness
- A belief that an iPod or radio is sending special messages intended just for them

Intense delusions might mean the person is suffering from a different illness, such as schizophrenia.

Q What is minor depression?

A *Minor depression*, or *dysthymia*, is like a smoldering major depression. Think of a fire, with embers not yet hot enough to ignite the logs above. A minor depression is like this, with symptoms from the recognized symptoms of major depression. The symptoms are bothersome and last at least 2 years at a low level, but usually not enough to disable the person. Yet the person affected doesn't feel well, and definitely doesn't enjoy life to the fullest. A person with minor depression is six times as likely to develop one or more full-blown episodes of major depression. Minor depression isn't so minor!

Q What is bipolar disorder?

A *Bipolar disorder* is a type of depression with two "poles"—one high and one low— that cycle back and forth (Table 2-2). These mood switches usually come on gradually and though it is rare, they can switch in rapid, dramatic fashion. Bipolar disorder is less common than the other types of depression, but it's just as serious and can progress to suicide or psychosis.

Table 2-2: Symptoms of Bipolar Disorder

All the symptoms from Table 2-1, plus:

- Decreased need for sleep, sometimes awake for days
- Many projects or things going at once, nothing meaningfully completed
- Grandiose thoughts, inflated sense of self and worth
- Increased energy, agitation, irritability
- Pressured speech, talking to excess
- Racing thoughts
- Inappropriate elation, expansiveness
- Increased sexual desire, possibly with inappropriate acting out and promiscuity
- Inappropriate social behaviors, like spending or gambling to excess
- Poor insight and judgment
- Hyper-religiosity

- In the depressed or low state, patients look like they have a major depression
- In the manic or high state, people have lots of excess energy, pressured speech, and racing thoughts

These symptoms aren't fleeting but are persistent and cause a person an obvious loss of function.

How does a medical professional know what kind of depression a person has?

Q

A

You may hear your doctor or mental health professional refer to your diagnosis using the term "DSM-4." This is the *Diagnostic and Statistical Manual, version 4,* the standard mental health diagnosis reference book. This manual contains all the signs and symptoms of the major mental disorders, including depression. These diagnoses are separated into groups, with codes for each diagnosis. A provider can only make a certain diagnosis if the required signs and symptoms are present. There are no blood tests or X-rays currently available to help make a diagnosis, so these strict rules for making diagnoses make sure that all medical professionals use the same treatment guidelines.

Consistent Diagnoses Ensure Consistent Treatments
By using the same criteria to diagnose depression, medical professionals are able to use the same treatment guidelines.

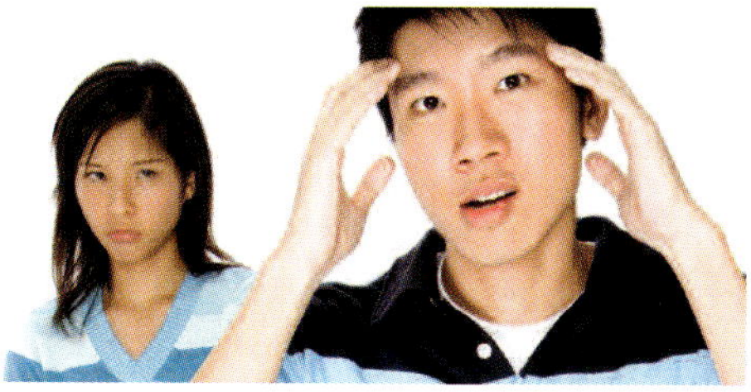

What Causes Depression?

Some people think that depression is a curse, a sign of weakness, or a sign of being weak in one's faith. It's none of these. Ultimately, depression is a medical illness that might have roots in one's family history, caused by personal stress (an illness nevertheless), or caused by complex imbalances in the brain's chemical activity but that can respond to treatment.

Depression Is an Illness
Ultimately, depression is a medical illness that might have roots in one's family history or personal stress, but which is an illness nevertheless.

Q

What are some of the most common causes of depression?

A

Depression probably isn't caused by any one thing, but comes about as a person is subjected to certain risk factors (Table 3-1). Some of the risk factors seem obvious, such as if you have suffered from depression in the past or if someone in your family has suffered from depression. Other risk factors are less obvious, such as not having social support—no family or friends with whom to share life's usual ups and downs.

Ultimately, the final common pathway for depression, whatever the cause, becomes a chemical imbalance in the brain.

Table 3-1: Risk Factors for Depression

- History of depression
- Family history of depression
- History of suicidal thinking or attempts
- Female gender
- Postpartum or perimenopausal period
- Serious medical illness
- Lack of social support
- High stress levels with family, job, finances, relationships
- History of or current alcohol or drug abuse

It All Comes Down to Chemicals
Ultimately, the final common pathway for depression is a chemical imbalance in the brain.

Q

My mother was diagnosed with depression. How likely is it that I will suffer from depression?

A

Having a blood relative—a parent or brother or sister—with depression can make you more susceptible to depression. However, it doesn't doom you to becoming depressed. Identical twins have the same genetic material, but if one becomes depressed, there is only a 60% chance that the other will become depressed. Figure 3-1 shows that there are many influences other than heredity that may predispose a person *to* depression—or even protect them *from* depression.

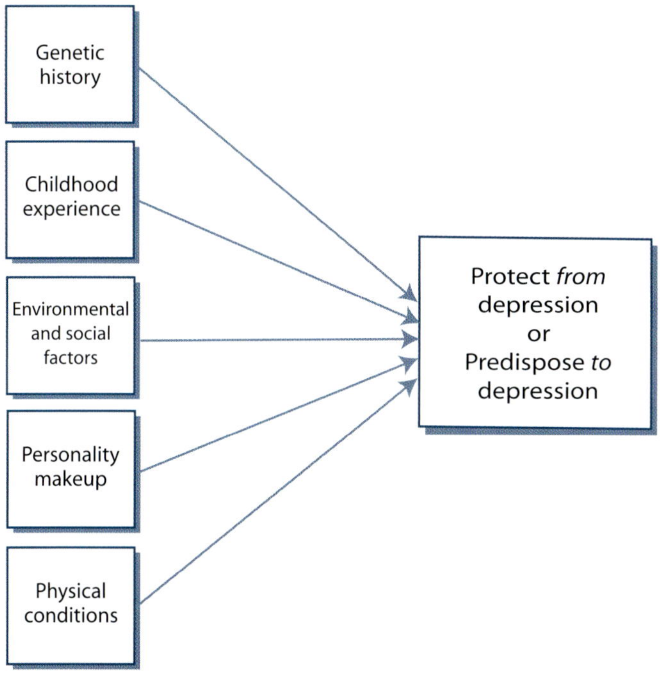

Figure 3-1. Protective or predisposing factors for depression.

Q

Why is it that women are more depressed than men?

A

Women become depressed twice as often as men, probably because they are cycling creatures, with hormones going up and down throughout their lives. They may also make less serotonin than men, a brain chemical important in regulating mood. One in eight women will develop depression within her lifetime, usually starting between the ages of 25 and 44. Women experience changes in hormone levels with the onset of their periods, during pregnancy, childbirth, the postpartum period, beginning and ending breastfeeding, the period leading to menopause (perimenopause), and menopause itself.

Q

So can a woman's depression be blamed on hormones?

A

Hormones are active in the brain, the seat of our thoughts and emotions, so it shouldn't be surprising that they can affect women's moods and behaviors. But there may also be social or cultural factors that influence female depression, such as the stresses of juggling work, homemaking, parenthood, and caring for aging parents.

Q

What's the relationship between stress and depression?

A

Stresses or major life changes (such as divorce, financial troubles, loss of a loved one) can bring on depression. People who have lost a parent or an important figure early in life may be particularly vulnerable.

Q

Can someone just be prone to depression?

A

Yes. Some people seem to have personalities predisposed to developing depression. They are the "Eeyores" of the world (Winnie the Pooh's sad donkey friend)—pessimists who look at life through dark glasses and lack the ability to soothe themselves when things get rough may not have the emotional reserves to deal with stress. In this group of patients, adding psychotherapy as part of the treatment plan is particularly important. Counseling can help change patterns of negative thinking and the tendency to see things as worse than they actually are.

Q

Can having another illness cause depression?

A

Yes. Some physical illnesses can lead to depression. Patients already stressed by coping with cancer, heart disease, stroke, or other illness can be blindsided by developing depression on top of these problems. Just because depression is understandable–"Anyone with cancer would be sad and depressed!"–doesn't mean there's nothing that can be done about it. Treating illness-associated depressions can often improve the illness itself.

Table 3-2 list some of the illnesses that are known to influence depression.

Q

Can medications that a person takes cause depression?

A

Yes. When patients are on medications and develop symptoms of depression, we must make sure that their "ills aren't from their pills" and rule out side effects from the medications as a cause. Some of the relationships between medicines and the appearance of symptoms of depression are quite strong (certain blood pressure medications, like reserpine or methyldopa, are known culprits). Others have a weaker connection, but common sense says that if a person without depression begins a new medication, and then develops depression without having other risk factors, perhaps the medication should be discontinued or changed. Don't ever stop any medication on your own–always consult with your doctor.

Q

Is it possible to have symptoms of depression—but not be depressed?

A

Yes. Some people develop symptoms of depression but don't have a psychiatric illness at all! These symptoms are the brain's way of alerting the body that it needs help—that something physical is wrong that needs attention.

It sounds like you're saying that depression can really strike anyone at any time. Is that true?

Essentially, yes. It doesn't discriminate. Depression is an equal opportunity illness, coming both in times of trouble and times of seeming peace. It affects people of all races, income levels, and educations. Depression is a nasty illness, sneaking in when people are least likely to be able to fight it off—after a death of a loved one, the loss of a job, or the onset of a serious illness. But it can also strike when things seem perfect, leading sufferers to ask, "Why should I feel sad? There's nothing wrong in my life!" This seems to make sense to the depressed person, but is like a person with cancer saying, "Why should I have cancer? There's nothing wrong in my life!"

Table 3-2: Illnesses and Medications Associated with Depression

Illnesses	**Medications**
Cancer, especially lung and pancreas	Antihypertensives/Blood pressure drugs
Heart disease	Catepres (Clonidine)
Chronic lung disease	Hydralazine
Diabetes	Methyldopa (Aldomet)
End-stage kidney disease/dialysis	Propranolol (Inderal)
Parkinson's disease	Reserpine (Hydergine)
Dementia	Cardiac drugs
Huntington's disease	Digitalis
Stroke	Procainamide
Seizure disorders or epilepsy	Lidocaine
Multiple sclerosis	Chemotherapy drugs
Chronic pain	Azathioprine (AZT)
Sleep disorders	Bleomycin
Rheumatoid arthritis	Vincristine (Oncovin)
Lupus	Steroids
HIV infection/AIDS	Histamine 2 receptor blockers
Syphilis	Cimetidine (Tagamet)
Lyme disease	Ranitidine (Zantac)
Viral infections, (influenza, mononucleosis, hepatitis)	Amantadine (Symmetrel)
Chronic fatigue syndrome	Phenytoin (Dilantin)
Endocrine diseases (thyroid, parathyroid, or adrenal glands)	Baclofen (Lioresal)
Vitamin B_{12} deficiency	Bromocriptine (Parlodel)
Substance use, abuse, or dependence	Isotretinoin (Accutane)
Other psychiatric disorders – anxiety disorders, eating disorders, personality disorders	
Note: Traumatic injuries and severe burns can also influence rates of depression	

CHAPTER FOUR

Who Suffers from Depression?

A wide cross-section of people suffer from depression, including women, men, children and adolescents, college students, the elderly, those with illnesses, and those with alcohol and addiction problems.

We'll discuss each of these groups of individuals in detail.

Women
Depression occurs more often in women, most likely because of the many shifts in hormone levels during their lives. So, it isn't surprising that women experience certain types of depression around times of hormonal activity.

Q

What's the link between menstruation and depression?

A

Premenstrual dysphoric disorder (or PMDD) (different from the milder premenstrual syndrome, or PMS) is a mood disorder related to the timing of a woman's menstrual cycle. This is more than just irritability or moodiness. It's a major depressive disorder that settles in a week or two before one's period and stops when the period begins. Symptoms include five or more of the following, with at least one of the first four:

- Increased, lasting anger or irritability; severe problems maintaining good relations with others
- Noticeable mood instability, short fuse
- Marked tension, anxiety, feeling "on edge"
- Noticeable depressed mood, negativity
- Decreased interest in usual activities
- Decreased attention and concentration
- Low energy, no "get-up-and-go"
- Decrease or increase in appetite, increase in cravings
- Decrease or increase in sleep
- Feeling overwhelmed, helpless, out of control
- Physical symptoms like breast swelling or tenderness, headaches, bloating, joint or muscle aches

Q

If I have many of these symptoms, does this mean I have PMDD?

A

To truly be diagnosed with PMDD, these symptoms should cause difficulties in functioning at home, school, or work, and need to persist for at least two menstrual cycles. You should have normal moods in between cycles. PMDD can occur in 3 to 5% of menstruating women. Many women have some symptoms that aren't disabling, so they're not considered to have the full-blown disorder.

How can pregnancy be related to depression?

Being pregnant is often considered to bring with it a sense of happiness and purpose, thus immunizing her from becoming depressed. In truth, pregnancy is an especially challenging time to maintain one's mental health. Women with a previous history of depression may find themselves suffering from a relapse during pregnancy, and women with no previous history of depression may find themselves similarly affected. Up to half a million women per year suffer from depression during pregnancy. Up to 15% of women will become depressed after delivery, a figure that rises to 50% if they had *post-partum depression* previously.

The Mental Challenges of Pregnancy

Up to half a million women per year suffer from depression during pregnancy. Up to 15% of women will become depressed after delivery, a figure that rises to 50% if they had *post-partum depression* previously.

If a woman develops depression during pregnancy, is she still at risk after the baby is born?

Yes. Women are especially vulnerable after their children are born. The hormonal and physical changes and the stress of caring for a new life can lead to what is known as *post-partum depression.* This is quite different from the syndrome known as "baby blues," which involve passing feelings of sadness and fatigue and fear, occurring in up to 50 to 80 % of women within a few days of delivery. These feelings go away on their own, usually after a week to 10 days. On the other hand, post-partum depression is a medical illness that requires aggressive treatment. It is the *most common* complication of childbirth.

After-Baby Depression

Post-partum depression is the most common complication of childbirth.

Hormones seem to influence many of the episodes of depression in women. Does menopause put a stop to that?

While it's true that women eventually stop their hormonal cycling, it's during the period of perimenopause (the time just before menopause) that these older women are at greatest risk for depression. Between 10 to 20% of women will suffer from depression during this time, and are especially at risk if they have a prior history of depression, a history of PMS, or particularly severe hot flashes that disturbs their sleep.

Men

Though it's more common in women, depression is certainly not exclusive to the female gender.

Is depression common in men?

Yes. Although women become depressed more than men, millions of men suffer from this illness every year, with men completing suicide four times as often as women.

Q Is it hard for men to admit depression?

A In general, yes. Perhaps because of a perception that depression is a weakness or a character flaw, men are less likely to admit to being depressed, seek out a doctor for treatment, and may attempt to mask depression by using alcohol or drugs to excess. Doctors and health care providers may be less likely to diagnose depression in a male patient, chalking up symptoms of fatigue, being "out-of-sorts" and may even blame symptoms on "workaholism."

Q What might it take for men to overcome the social stigma of depression?

A Possibly it will be when men understand that some of the most famous men in history suffered from (and overcame) depression (for example, Abraham Lincoln and Winston Churchill). Then, more inroads can be made in successfully diagnosing and treating this illness in the male population. The National Institute of Mental Health (part of the National Institutes of Health) is trying to get the word out through their "Real Men, Real Depression" campaign. You'll find more information on how to get information from the Institute in Chapter 11.

Even the Highest Office Isn't Immune

"I am now the most miserable man living. If what I feel were equally distributed to the whole human family there would not be one cheerful face on earth. Whether I shall ever be better, I cannot tell; I awfully forebode I shall not. To remain as I am is impossible. I must die or be better, it appears to me."

—Abraham Lincoln

Children and Adolescents

Depression in children and adolescents is just as serious as in older patients, and only recently has become a focus of clinical attention.

Q So children can actually be depressed?

A Yes. Nearly 3 million children and adolescents suffer from depression every year. Also, depression starts earlier now than in the past. If untreated, these young patients can go on to develop problems with alcohol and drug addiction and eating disorders. Female patients are at risk for adolescent pregnancy. Pediatric depression can kill its young victims as easily as adult depression can. Over half of untreated youngsters will attempt suicide; about 5% will be successful at their attempt.

"The burden of suffering by children with mental health needs and their families has created a health crisis in this country. Growing numbers of children [and adolescents] are suffering needlessly because their emotional, behavioral, and developmental needs are not being met by the very institutions and systems that were created to take care of them".

—Surgeon General's Conference on Children's Mental Health (2001)

Q What are the signs of depression in children and adolescents?

A The symptoms can be very hard to sort out, as children do go through "phases" as part of normal childhood and adolescent development. Table 4-1 lists some of the common symptoms.

Signs of depression can be especially hard to spot in adolescents, as moodiness is part of being a teenager, and the teen-aged brain is still growing and developing. Teens are trying to find their place in the world and are re-negotiating their roles with parents, teachers, and friends. Nevertheless, concerned parents shouldn't hesitate to speak with their children's teachers or school counselors and take them to their pediatricians for diagnosis and treatment, if needed. Drug and alcohol abuse must also be ruled out.

Table 4-1. Symptoms of Depression in Children and Adolescents

Both genders	Refusing to go to school Pretending to be ill Worrying a parent might die Not allowing the parent to go out of his or her sight Sullenness Irritability Exhibiting uncharacteristic bad behaviors at school Plummeting grades
Girls	Increased anxiety Symptoms of eating disorders Cutting themselves
Boys	Increased aggressive behaviors or acting out

What advice do you have for the parent or caregiver of a depressed child or teen?

Q

A

The best advice is that any child with depression needs to be closely and carefully monitored by their health care professionals, especially early in the course of treatment, when suicide risk is greatest. If children or adolescents seem to be more irritable or have an increase in symptoms after medications are prescribed or changed, call your pediatrician or mental health care provider right away. We must do all we can to get these young people well and enhance their chances of remaining well into adulthood.

College Students

College-age students are an interesting group of people to consider, as they are exactly at the age when many mental illnesses begin.

Are college-age students prone to depression?

Q

A

As the age of onset of depression starts earlier and earlier, many students are entering college already ill. When you couple an ill student with the stresses of being newly independent, away from home for the first time, coping with academic and financial stressors, and forming and keeping new relationships, you have a recipe for disaster. Many students won't admit or seek help out of shame or fear of being shunned by friends or social groups. They may not go to their professors, from whom they might need to obtain recommendations for jobs or graduate school in the future. Some students turn to drugs and alcohol. They suffer in silence—and some may die from their silence.

Recipe for Disaster

When you couple an ill student with the stresses of being newly independent, away from home for the first time, coping with academic and financial stressors, and forming and keeping new relationships, you have a recipe for disaster.

Q

What can be done to help people in this age group?

A

Depression in this age bracket demands a higher level of awareness on the part of college professors and staff in detecting and referring depressed students to treatment. Campus-wide health fairs should include education on depression, information on stress and how to manage it, free depression screenings, and easy access to counseling.

Those already medically ill

Whether the illness causes the depression or the depression affects the illness, the outcome is the same: the depressed, ill person now has two afflictions to deal with.

Q

How can one tell if it's depression or the illness causing the symptoms of depression?

A

It can be difficult. Treating depression in medically ill patients can be challenging, as many of the symptoms of medical illness—sleeping problems, low energy, poor appetite—are the same as the main symptoms of depression. These warning signs are often minimized by patients and family members who think that feeling depressed is normal for people dealing with serious illnesses. A doctor should carefully look at the ill patient's mindset and patterns of thinking to see if the patient is feeling hopeless or helpless to the point of wishing to die, or if they have lost hope in a situation that may still point to recovery.

Illness Doesn't Have To Mean Depression

Many warning signs of depression—sleeping problems, low energy, poor appetite—are often minimized by patients and family members who think that feeling depressed is normal for people dealing with serious illnesses.

Q

Can depression cause illness or make an illness worse?

A

Yes. Untreated depression can lead to illness or make pre-existing illnesses worse. For example:

- Depression can worsen heart disease and even cause early death. After a heart attack, 40 to 65% of patients will become depressed, and have a 3 to 4 times better chance of dying within the next 6 months.
- Adult onset diabetics have a 1 in 4 chance of being depressed, which can lead to poor blood sugar control.
- Depression seems to be a risk factor for stroke, and post-stroke patients have an incidence of depression after stroke ranging from 10 to 35%. If untreated, slows recovery and increases risk of death.

To complicate matters, depressed patients are less likely to follow medical instructions, making it difficult to treat their medical condition.

It seems likely that the terminally ill can become depressed. Is this true?

It's very true, and treating severe depression in terminally ill patients needs special mention. These patients can benefit from the boost that treating their depression might give them, but they may not have 4 to 8 weeks to wait for full effectiveness of an antidepressant. Most commonly, psychostimulant (mood-elevating) medications are given, such as methylphenidate (Ritalin) or dextroamphetamine (Dexedrine). These medications can boost energy, appetite, and the ability to concentrate, work quickly if they are going to be effective, and are very well tolerated. *Electroconvulsive therapy* (discussed more in Chapter 6) can sometimes be used in these patients to give them some relief after one or two treatments.

The Elderly

Just as with the younger population, depression knows no age restrictions.

Is depression common in older people?

Yes, depression is common, but it's *not* a normal part of aging. As with any other age, depression is an illness that causes terrible suffering in the person and those who love them. It's very treatable, but the doctor or mental health care provider must be alert to the fact that depression can present differently in older patients. Often these patients are fiercely proud and regard depression as a weakness or a sign of being "crazy." They will rarely voluntarily ask for help.

In Depression Denial

Older, depressed patients are often fiercely proud and regard depression as a weakness or a sign of being "crazy." They will rarely voluntarily ask for help.

Is the older depressed person so different than someone younger who is depressed?

Depression in the elderly may sometimes present differently. Symptoms may look like physical symptoms—constipation, unrelenting chronic pain, or problems with concentration or memory. Depressed elders may withdraw from things that previously gave them much pleasure, saying they don't feel well enough or have the energy. The rate of depression in nursing home residents can run as high as 25%. Doctors also need to make sure that an elder's "ills aren't from their pills," as older patients tend to be on a larger number of medications, some of which can have depression as a side effect.

Do the same reasons contribute to depression in an older person as in a younger person?

Many things can contribute to the start of a depression in an older patient. It can be a recurrence of depression experienced previously, or can appear for the first time. Society sometimes believes, however, that with all the usual losses old age brings, "Anyone would be depressed." Table 4-2 lists several of the reasons for depression in this age group. Depression that appears for the first time should prompt the doctor to look for physical problems like a hidden cancer or undiagnosed thyroid disease. Chronic or serious illness can also kick off a geriatric depression.

Do elderly depressed patients suffer any special risks?

Yes. Sadly, fewer than 10% of depressed elders seek help. The risk of completing suicide is highest in the elderly and they generally prefer more violent means of ending their lives, such as self-inflicted gunshot wounds or jumping out of high windows.

Table 4-2: What Causes Depression in the Elderly

Illnesses	Late Life Losses
Cancer	Spouse
Parkinson's disease	Friends
Chronic obstructive pulmonary disease (COPD)	Job
Heart disease	House
Stroke	Eyesight
Diabetes with complications	Hearing
End-stage renal disease	Vitality
Dementia	

The Alcoholic/Addicted Patient

This population of depressed patients is particularly challenging to diagnose and treat. Many patients will see a doctor but are afraid to disclose their drug or alcohol problems out of a sense of shame or embarrassment or fear of legal consequences. They may report symptoms of depression or anxiousness and say that they are using alcohol or drugs to "self-medicate" because it relaxes them, helps them sleep, or numbs their pain.

Q

Do drug and alcohol use complicate depression?

A

Yes. In fact, doctors must take a careful history to solve the "chicken or the egg" puzzle—which came first: the depression or the addiction? This is very important, as alcohol and drugs can *cause* depression and anxiety. If someone began abusing drugs and alcohol *before* they began to have psychiatric symptoms—and if it can be shown that the depression goes away when the drinking or drug abuse stops—then the depression most likely will go away when the addiction is treated. No treatment (antidepressant or psychotherapy) will be effective until a person is clean and sober.

Q

Is it possible for a person to be depressed without it having anything to do with their drug or alcohol abuse?

A

Yes. Some patients with depression can have drug and alcohol problems independent of their psychiatric illness. In particular, many patients with bipolar disorder abuse alcohol and drugs. Treatments for the psychiatric disorder must proceed. But, again, it likely can't be fully effective until the addictions are addressed.

Addiction and Depression

For people to get well emotionally, they must be well physically—and ignoring problems with drugs and alcohol prevents patients from achieving their best physical and mental health.

CHAPTER FIVE

How is Depression Diagnosed?

If you suspect that you are experiencing a depression or that someone you love is experiencing a depression, the first step is to see a doctor for a thorough history and physical exam.

First Things First
If you suspect that you are experiencing a depression or that someone you love is experiencing a depression, the first step is to see a doctor for a thorough history and physical exam.

Q
A

What will the doctor look for?

First, the doctor will want to take a thorough history. A good history requires the patient and those who may be with him or her for support to be candid and truthful (Table 5-1). The doctor may want to know things like:

- When did the symptoms start?
- Were there any stressors that came before the depression?
- Has the patient had problems with depression before?
- If so, what was the treatment, and was it successful?
- Has any family member struggled with depression and if so, what treatment was successful for him or her?
- Has the patient had thoughts of suicide or psychotic thoughts?
- Does the patient have any problems with drugs or alcohol?

Table 5-1: Diagnosing Depression: What Your Doctor Will Do

- Take a thorough history
- Perform a mental status exam
- Order lab tests or perform a physical examination to rule out any other illness
- Recommend an antidepressant and/or refer you to a mental health provider

Q

Are the answers to these questions enough to diagnose depression?

A

No. A good evaluation also includes a mental status exam. During this exam, the patient is asked about mood symptoms or problems with thinking, and is also tested on measures of attention, concentration, memory, and rationality. All of these can be negatively affected by depression.

Q

Will the doctor perform any physical tests?

A

Perhaps. He or she may want to order some lab work or X-rays to make sure there is no underlying physical disease causing the symptoms. However, there isn't a specific lab test or X-ray to diagnose depression!

Q

What if the doctor finds no physical problems?

A

If everything else is ruled out, your doctor may want to start you on an antidepressant, may refer you to a mental health provider for counseling, or may refer you to a psychiatrist for medication and treatment.

Q

Is there any way I can diagnose depression myself?

A

On the Internet, good screening tests are available that can help you or a loved one decide if the situation warrants a professional evaluation. Chapter 11 lists some reputable Internet sites that can help you. However, screening tests don't take the place of a professional evaluation. If someone is depressed and suicidal, they must seek professional help immediately (Table 5-2).

Table 5-2: You Think You're Depressed: Now What?

- Self-screen
- Contact your primary care doctor
- Follow through with mental health professional, if advised
- Be honest!

Take the Test

You can self-perform a screening test, but these don't take the place of a professional evaluation.

Q

Chapter 3 mentioned a chemical imbalance as the ultimate cause of depression. No blood test can reveal this?

A

Unfortunately, no. Even if, as we suspect, depression is ultimately caused by a disturbance of chemicals in the brain, there is still no blood test to determine what these imbalances are.

CHAPTER SIX

How is Depression Treated?

Depression is very treatable. People don't have to suffer in silence. The earlier and more aggressively depression is detected and treated, the less likely it will have chronic, disabling effects. Types of treatment vary by case and include:

- Physical (medications)
- Psychological (counseling)
- Complementary (something you can do or take *in addition to* medication and/or counseling) and
- Alternative (something you can do or take *instead of* medication and/or counseling)

We'll discuss each of these in depth.

Don't Suffer in Silence
Depression is very treatable. People don't have to suffer in silence.

Going All the Way
The aim for treatment isn't better, but *best;* not a bit more well, but *all the way well.*

Are most depressed patients treated as outpatients?

Q

A

Yes. People who can care for themselves and who aren't psychotic or suicidal can usually be treated as outpatients with antidepressants and/or psychotherapy. Either treatment alone can be effective, but a combined medication/psychotherapy approach is the best path to getting all the way well.

What if the depression is severe?

Q

A

If someone is acutely suicidal or psychotic, it's best for them to be treated in a hospital. There, professionals can monitor their safety and provide aggressive treatment. Some are afraid of this option, thinking about the negative stereotypes of psychiatric wards depicted in old movies or novels. The modern psychiatric hospital is much like any other hospital, with the emphasis on emotional treatments and therapies rather than physical ones.

Do the severely depressed have to check into a hospital?

Q

A

Not all the time. There are "partial hospitals" for people who are severely ill but who can remain safe and care for themselves. These are intensive outpatient programs where someone can go a half day to one full day 3 to 5 days a week, but still live at home and maintain a daily routine.

Q Who can treat depression?

A Several professionals are qualified to treat depression, and these are listed in Table 6-1.

- Most general practitioners are familiar with antidepressants and can prescribe treatment after an appropriate work-up. This is the best place to start because a doctor can rule out physical causes of depression. These doctors can make a referral, if needed.
- Psychiatrists are medical doctors with special training in mental health who can both prescribe medications and provide psychotherapy.
- Psychologists and licensed social workers can also make a diagnosis and provide counseling, but can't prescribe medication.

Many patients participate in a split-treatment model. Their family doctor or psychiatrist provides the medications and a therapist provides the counseling.

Table 6-1: Therapists for Depression: Who Are They?
• Psychiatrist (MD/DO)
• Psychologist (PhD or licensed)
• Licensed social worker

Physical Treatments for Depression

The physical treatments for depression include:

- Medications
- Electroconvulsive therapy
- Vagal Nerve Stimulation
- Repetitive Transcranial Magnetic Stimulation and
- Light therapy

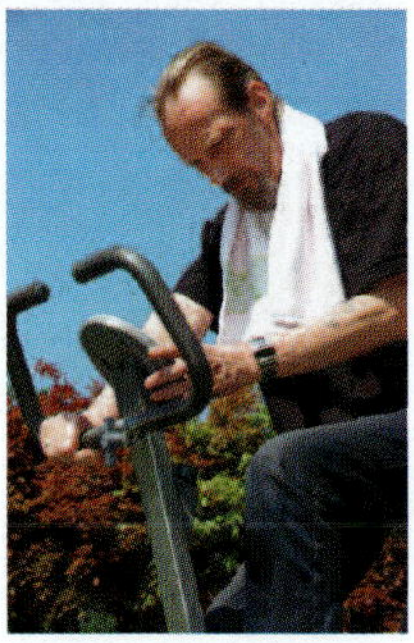

We'll discuss each of these in depth.

Medications

Q Is medication absolutely necessary to treat depression?

A Milder forms of depression may respond to some non-medical approaches to treatment (described later) or to psychotherapy alone. But most depression will be controlled faster and for longer periods of time if medications are also used. Several classes of antidepressants are available. How they work and what side effects they may cause are different. These are described in Table 6-2.

Table 6-2: Classes of Antidepressant Medications

What they are; Brand Name (generic name)	**How they work**	**Side effects**	**Handling side effects**
SSRIs			
• Prozac, Sarafem, Prozac weekly (fluoxetine) • Zoloft (sertraline) • Paxil, Pexeva, Paxil CR (paroxetine) • Celexa (citalopram) • Lexapro (escitalopram)	Increases the level of the brain chemical serotonin	Headache, mild nausea, diarrhea, dry mouth, jitteriness, insomnia, weight gain (paroxetine), fatigue, and sexual dysfunction Consider your sexual functioning before starting any medication. If sexual functioning or desire worsens after starting an SSRI, but other depressive symptoms are getting better, it could be an SSRI side effect. Do not use within 2 weeks of stopping an MAOI (defined later in this table).	• Start with a low dose and increase slowly. • Take with food to avoid upset stomach. • If medications activate you, take them in the morning. • If medications sedate you, take them at bedtime. • If sexual side effects don't improve with time, a small dose of another antidepressant called Wellbutrin (buproprion) may help. • With the exception of Prozac (fluoxetine), most medications (especially Paxil/Pexeva (paroxetine)) need to be tapered gradually to avoid dizziness, GI upset, "pins and needles" feelings in the limbs, insomnia, and vivid dreaming. These symptoms will go away within a few days of discontinuing the medication.

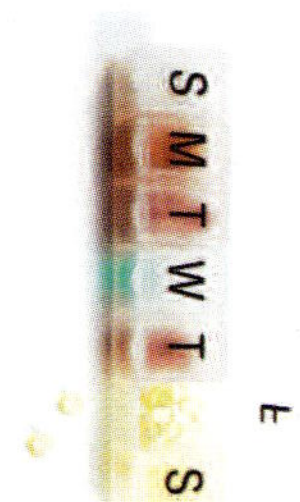

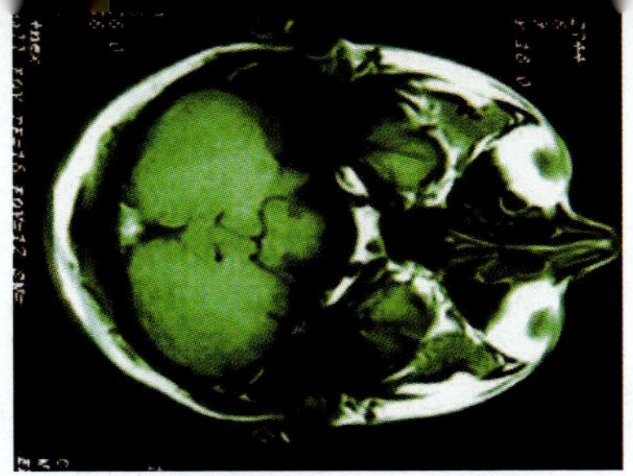

Table 6-2: Classes of Antidepressant Medications (continued)

What they are; Brand Name (generic name)	How they work	Side effects	Handling side effects
Other antidepressants			
Wellbutrin SR, XL (bupropion SR, XL) (also marketed as Zyban, for use in smoking cessation)	Increases levels of the brain chemicals norepinephrine and dopamine	Jitteriness, dry mouth, nausea, insomnia, headache, decreased appetite, dizziness. Does not tend to increase weight and may cause mild weight loss. Tends not to affect sexual appetite and performance and may improve them. Should not be used in patients who also have a seizure disorder, or a history or active case of bulimia or anorexia nervosa (both eating disorders). Should not be used in patients who have stopped using alcohol or benzodiazepine sedatives suddenly, like Valium or Xanax, as this increases the risk of seizures. Do not use within 2 weeks of stopping an MAOI.	• All should decrease with time, and can be lessened or avoided by starting with a low dose and going up slowly. • Suck on sugarless candies or drink no-calorie fluids to relieve dry mouth. • Try taking with food if nausea is an issue. • If taking the SR form and sleep is a problem, take the second dose at supper, not at bedtime.

Table 6-2: Classes of Antidepressant Medications (continued)

What they are; Brand Name (generic name)	**How they work**	**Side effects**	**Handling side effects**
Serzone (nefazodone)		Only the generic (nefazodone) is still available in the United States. Serzone was withdrawn from the U.S. market in response to declining sales and a concern of a very small rate of liver failure in patients.	
Desyrel (trazodone)	Increases levels of the brain chemical serotonin	Drowsiness, dizziness when standing up suddenly, headache at higher doses. This agent is so sedating at antidepressant doses that it's mainly used as a sleep aid, often along with some of the more activating antidepressants. One in 6,000 male patients may experience persistent and painful penile erection (*priapism*).	• Take at bedtime to take advantage of its sedating effect. • Priapism is considered a medical emergency, so men experiencing a prolonged erection lasting more than 1 hour should proceed to the nearest ER, where an antidote can be given.
Effexor IR, XR (venlafaxine)	Inhibits levels of the brain chemicals serotonin and norepinephrine	Nausea, increase in blood pressure at higher doses, sweating, dry mouth, constipation, headache, fatigue, insomnia, and sexual dysfunction. Do not use within 2 weeks of stopping an MAOI.	• Take with food to decrease upset stomach. • Start at low dose and increase gradually to decrease nausea. • Do not stop abruptly to avoid dizziness and anxiety.

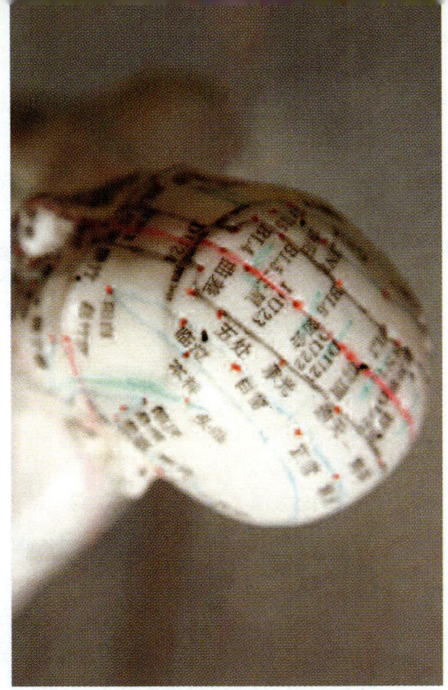

Table 6-2: Classes of Antidepressant Medications (continued)

What they are; Brand Name (generic name)	**How they work**	**Side effects**	**Handling side effects**
Cymbalta (duloxetine)	Inhibits levels of the brain chemicals serotonin and norepinephrine	Nausea, dry mouth, constipation, fatigue, jitteriness, headache, insomnia, sexual dysfunction, increased sweating. Should not be used in patients with liver failure.	See TCA section, below.
Remeron (mirtazapine)	Enhances activity of the brain chemicals norepinephrine and serotonin	Drowsiness, weight gain, dry mouth. Very rarely can cause decrease in white cell count which can affect the body's ability to fight off infections.	• Take the dose at bedtime. • Use with caution in overweight patients. • Oddly enough, side effects may diminish with higher doses of the drug.

Table 6-2: Classes of Antidepressant Medications (continued)

What they are; Brand Name (generic name)	How they work	Side effects	Handling side effects
TCAs (Tricyclic antidepressants)			
• Anafranil (clomipramine) • Elavil (amitriptyline) • Pamelor, Aventyl (nortriptyline) • Norpramin (desipramine) • Sinequan (doxepin) • Vivactil (protriptyline) • Surmontil (trimipramine) • Tofranil (imipramine) • Asendin (amoxapine)	Affects the brain chemicals norepinephrine and serotonin in varying amounts.	Dry mouth, constipation, problems urinating, blurry vision, dizziness when standing up abruptly, daytime drowsiness, sexual performance problems, weight gain (amitriptyline, doxepin, imipramine). Interactions with certain heart medicines, especially ones used to regulate heartbeat. Not for use in patients with narrow-angle glaucoma. Do not use within 2 weeks of stopping an MAOI.	• Sugarless hard candies or sugar-free fluids will help with dry mouth and constipation. • Ingest adequate bulk and fiber in the diet; mild exercise will help with depression and constipation. • Stand up slowly from a sitting or lying position to help with dizziness. • If medications cause drowsiness, take most (or all) of the daily dose at bedtime or after dinner. • Use caution while driving or doing tasks which require alertness until you get used to the medication, or drowsiness goes away. • If side effects do not go away in time, or if depressive symptoms do not appear to lift, consider a medication change. • Doses may need to be halved in the elderly.

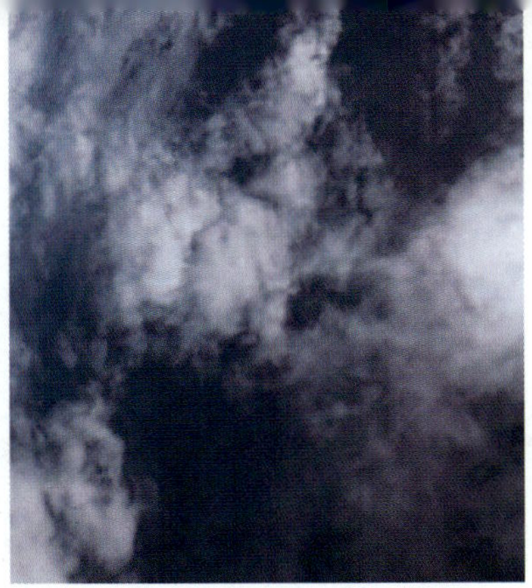

Table 6-2: Classes of Antidepressant Medications (continued)

What they are; Brand Name (generic name)	How they work	Side effects	Handling side effects
MAOIs (Monoamine oxidase inhibitors)			
•Nardil (phenelzine) •Parnate (tranylcypromine) •Marplan (isocarboxazid)	Affect the enzymes that break down certain brain chemicals, making more of them available to the brain	Insomnia, dizziness when suddenly standing up, weight gain, sexual dysfunction, risk of hypertensive crisis (a dangerous marked rise in blood pressure) if exposed to tyramine or certain drugs.	•Don't take too close to bedtime. •Take time standing from a sitting or lying position. •Avoid tyramine-containing foods and drugs (see Table 6-3).
• EMSAM (selegiline transdermal) This new treatment will most likely be used if more traditional oral medications are not effective.	This is not an oral medication but a patch that is placed on dry skin on the upper body, upper arm, or upper thigh area, allowing the medicine to be directly absorbed into the patient's bloodstream for 24 hours. One patch is used per day.	Irritation at the site of the patch, headache, mild stomach upset, and mild sleep disturbance	• At highest doses, must avoid tyramine-containing foods and drugs (see Table 6-3).

Table 6-2: Classes of Antidepressant Medications (continued)

What they are; Brand Name (generic name)	How they work	Side effects	Handling side effects
Medications for bipolar disorder			
• Eskalith, Lithane, Lithobid (lithium)	Not yet known	Diarrhea, weight gain, acne, mild hand tremor, decrease in thyroid gland function. Generally should not be used in pregnancy. Many drug-drug interactions so check with physician or psychiatrist if a new medication is added. Maintain good fluid intake as dehydration can cause lithium toxicity.	• Different forms of lithium may be tolerated better. • To combat weight gain, exercise and watch diet. • Take with food to minimize stomach upset. • If possible, take lower dose to see if tremor improves, or try a beta blocker like Inderal (propranolol)
• Depakote, Depekene (valproic acid)	Not yet known	Diarrhea, weight gain, mild tremor, sedation, inflammation of the liver or pancreas (hepatitis or pancreatitis), or abnormal blood count. Should generally not be used in pregnancy. Many drug-drug interactions so check with your physician or psychiatrist if a new medication is added.	• Different forms of valproic acid may be tolerated better. • To combat weight gain, exercise and watch diet. • Take with food to minimize stomach upset.
• Lamictal (lamotrigine)	Not yet known	Upset stomach, rash. One rare form of rash can be very severe and life-threatening, so report any skin change to the doctor.	• Start at low dose and increase slowly to avoid most side effects. • Take with food or milk to avoid stomach upset.

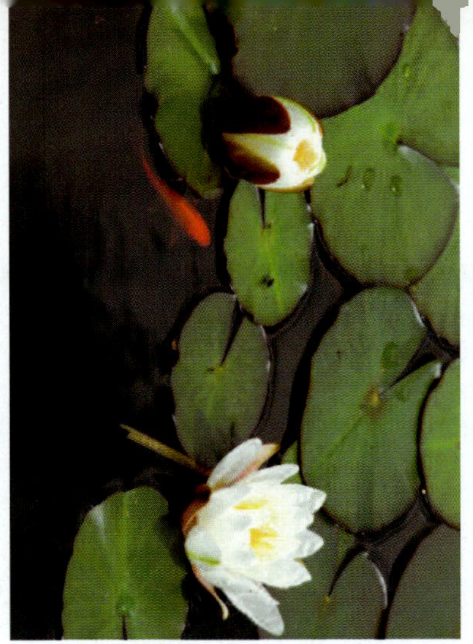

Table 6-2: Classes of Antidepressant Medications (continued)

What they are; Brand Name (generic name)	**How they work**	**Side effects**	**Handling side effects**
• Topamax (topiramate)	Not yet known	Weight loss, fuzzy thinking, "pins and needles" feelings in the limbs. Very rarely can result in kidney stones and/or worsening of glaucoma	• Monitor weight. • Use lowest dose possible for maximum effect. • Maintain fluid intake. • If fuzzy thinking does not go away with time another medication may need to be considered.
• Carbamazepine (tegretol)	Not yet known	Dizziness, drowsiness, rash, low blood sodium level, rare decrease in blood cells. Should generally not be used in pregnancy. Many drug-drug interactions so check with your physician or psychiatrist if a new medication is added.	• Start with a low dose and increase slowly.

Table 6-3: Tyramine-free Diet

Avoid these items if you are prescribed an MAOI:

Food Sources	Medications
Soy sauce	Dextromethorphan (found in many cough medicines)
Tofu	Decongestants
Sauerkraut	Certain anticonvulsants, including carbamazepine or oxcarbazepine (Tegretol, Trileptal)
Fava beans	Certain pain relievers, including tramadol (Ultram), meperidine (Demerol), Methadone, and propoxyphene (Darvon)
Aged meats	SSRIs
Pickled or cured meats and fishes	St John's Wort
Fermented fruit	Certain antidepressants, including nefazodone, venlafaxine (Effexor IR, XR), duloxetine (Cymbalta), and mirtazapine (Remeron)
Meat tenderizer	Tricyclic antidepressants (TCAs)
Red wines	Buspirone (BuSpar) (anti-anxiety)
Beer	Cyclobenzaprine (Flexeril) (muscle relaxant)
Aged cheeses	
Yogurt	
Concentrated yeast or meat extracts	

How does medication work on depression?

There is still so much about the brain we don't know, but it appears that antidepressants may work by affecting the function of certain chemicals in the brain. These chemicals include serotonin, norepinephrine, and dopamine.

How Antidepressants Work

Antidepressants work by affecting the function of certain brain chemicals, including serotonin, norepinephrine, and dopamine.

How long does it take for medication to "kick in"?

All antidepressants take 4 to 6 weeks for full effectiveness, and should never be stopped abruptly. Some symptoms –like disturbed sleep or low energy– may be helped within the first week. Patients should *not* take extra medication thinking that it might help the depression go away faster. It's important to give the medications a chance to work and to call your doctor with any questions.

If I take an antidepressant and begin to feel relief from the symptoms, how long do I need to keep taking it?

Once you are feeling all the way well, you should stick with the antidepressant for at least 6 to 12 months in order to make absolutely certain that the depression has been forced into remission. Some people with risk factors for chronic depression need to take medications indefinitely. If this is the first episode of depression, most doctors will recommend staying on the antidepressant for at least 6 months. If it's a second episode, stay on the antidepressant at least 1 year. If it's the third episode (or more), most doctors would recommend staying on the antidepressant indefinitely.

Q

What if the antidepressant prescribed doesn't seem to work?

A

Sometimes people may not seem to improve on the first prescribed antidepressant. If this occurs, several options can be considered (Table 6-4).

Table 6-4: Depression Treatment: If at First You Don't Succceed…

- Ask your doctor to check medication level to see if it is high enough
- Ask your doctor to make sure diagnosis is correct
- Avoid complicating factors such as drug and alcohol abuse
- Add psychotherapy
- Switch to different antidepressant medication
- Consider electroconvulsant therapy if it is urgent to obtain improvement

Q

I've heard of so many different antidepressants. How do doctors know which one to prescribe?

A

All antidepressants work, so picking one to try should be individualized to the person as some work for certain patients and not others. All antidepressants can also have side effects, so one should be selected with these in mind. For example, an overweight patient probably won't do well on a medication known to cause weight gain. But this medication might be a godsend for someone so ravaged by depression that they lost 30 pounds and have no appetite. Also, if a person or their family member previously did well on a certain medication, that might be the one to select.

Q

Once an antidepressant is prescribed, is that the only one that is ever prescribed?

A

Sometimes it's necessary to change the antidepressant, but some antidepressants might not work as well in certain patients. Also, there's an element of risk in changing medications, as you'll see in some of the side effect information (see Table 6-2).

Q

Do most insurance plans pay for antidepressants?

A

Most insurers now have "formularies" or approved listings for certain medications. It's wise to make sure that the antidepressant selected is on your insurance formulary, or that it comes in a generic form (if insurance isn't available) or you might find it difficult to pay for needed drugs. Most treatment failures happen because people don't stay on medications long enough, or take doses that aren't high enough.

Q

Can I get addicted to antidepressants?

A

No. Antidepressants aren't "happy pills," or "uppers." They aren't addictive or habit-forming, though most need to be tapered gradually before being stopped.

Q

Is there anything I should avoid if I'm taking an antidepressant?

A

Yes. You shouldn't take antidepressants with drugs or alcohol, as these will absolutely reduce their effectiveness and in some cases may cause severe side effects.

Do antidepressants have side effects?

Q A

Most antidepressants do have some side effects but these usually go away in time. People may find them annoying, but not serious. Side effects usually begin early on in treatment, as a person's body adjusts to it. Classes of antidepressants and their most common side effects are listed in Table 6-2. It's important to keep taking the medication even if side effects occur—you should call a doctor if you are concerned about them or if they persist or worsen.

What are the different types of antidepressants?

Q A

There are several classes of antidepressants:

- **SSRIs (selective serotonin re-uptake inhibitors).** SSRIs are the most commonly used antidepressants. They are fairly easy to dose and, most importantly, are less likely to cause death after an overdose.
- **TCAs (tricyclic antidepressants)** and **MAOIs (monoamine oxidase inhibitors).** TCAs and MAOIs are some of the oldest antidepressants (used exclusively from the 1950s to the 1980s), but are used less frequently today because of side effects and toxicities, including death in the event of overdose. Both are still used today for patients whose illness hasn't responded to newer medications.
- **Medications for bipolar disorder.** For many years, lithium has been the mainstay of treatment. It's been used since the 1950s and is relatively cheap and effective. Lithium isn't for everyone, however, and for those who can't tolerate it, there are alternatives. Most people with bipolar disorder require more than one medication, psychotherapy, and close monitoring by their health care team to get all the way well. The names of these antidepressants, how they work, and their side effects are in Table 6-2.

Medications in Special Populations

Children and Adolescents

Are antidepressants safe for children and adolescents?

Q A

Although there are some safety concerns about the use of antidepressants in this population, they can be lifesaving, especially when combined with psychotherapy. Prozac (fluoxetine) is the only U.S. Food and Drug Administration-approved antidepressant for pediatric depression. Other SSRIs may be appropriately used even though not yet FDA-approved for a particular use.

Recently, the FDA placed a *black box warning* on all antidepressants concerning their use in children and adolescents, noting that they can increase the frequency of suicidal thoughts and behaviors. A *black box warning* is a warning on a prescription drug label that describes the increased risk of suicide in pediatric patients and emphasizes the need to closely monitor patients taking them.

Are children on antidepressants more likely to commit suicide or behave dangerously?

Q A

To date, there has *not* been an increase in completed suicides in children and adolescents treated with antidepressants. There were no actual suicides in the FDA study that led to the black box warning, and this study looked at over 4,400 patients taking antidepressants. In fact, a recent study showed that the use of SSRIs in this population led to a *decrease* in the adolescent suicide rate of more than 25%! Yet parents, worried about sensationalized media reports about the small number of children who have gone "off" while on these medications and committed irrational violent acts toward others, have been increasingly hesitant to use medications in their children. Because of this, millions of children and adolescents are left untreated or partially treated.

Q

Is there anything we can do for depressed youngsters that doesn't involve medication?

A

As with adults, the best care for most children and adolescents combines medications plus psychotherapy. Family therapy and peer support groups can also be invaluable. In 2004, a study called TADS (Treatment for Adolescents with Depression Study) showed that Prozac (fluoxetine) plus psychotherapy got more depressed teens well than either treatment alone or from a placebo (a pill having no effect, but which a person believes or is led to believe will help their symptoms). Those patients also showed the greatest decrease in suicidal thinking.

Q

Pregnant and Nursing Women

Can pregnant women take antidepressants?

A

There is ongoing controversy about the use of antidepressants during pregnancy. Risks exist both with and without medication.

With no medication:

- Women with untreated depression can negatively influence their babies by not caring for themselves adequately or by abusing drugs or alcohol.
- Untreated depression can cause children to be born prematurely or with low birth weight, with symptoms of irritability, fussiness, lethargy, and decreased motor tone.

With medication:

- The FDA has issued an advisory about using SSRIs in the third trimester of pregnancy, noting that the newborns could be at risk for toxicity or withdrawal symptoms (tremor, fussiness, problems eating or sleeping, rigidity). The good news appears to be that no studies have yet shown long-term problems in these infants, who made full recoveries within 2 weeks.
- The FDA has issued an advisory specifically warning about the use of Paxil (paroxetine) in pregnancy, noting a small but statistically significant increase in an abnormality involving the heart in babies born to mothers who used Paxil in the first 3 months of their pregnancy. Other-large scale studies didn't report this increased risk.

Ultimately the decision is a careful one, balancing the needs of the two patients–mother and baby–as well as the risks and benefits of treatment vs. no treatment. If mom has had severe problems with depression, the benefit to both her and baby in continuing the medication may well outweigh the small risk to the infant.

Q

What about once the baby is born? Is it safe for new mothers with post-partum depression to take antidepressants?

A

Further complicating issues in post-partum depression is the issue of breastfeeding. A baby still in the womb can't help but be exposed to the mother's medications. A nursing mother also exposes her baby to medications. This situation is problematic: a mother feeling badly enough with her symptoms, now is caught between her welfare and that of her baby. The benefits of breastfeeding are well-known: better bonding between mom and baby, increased immunity against infections passed from mom to baby, and (practically speaking) a built-in safe source of nutrition for the baby available 24/7.

Q

How dangerous is it for the antidepressant to get into breast milk?

A

SSRIs are the class of antidepressants with the most data in breastfeeding. Most studies show amounts of the mother's antidepressant in her breast milk to be nearly undetectable, with the exception of Prozac (fluoxetine), which stays in the body longer than others. One study showed that about 5% of babies breastfed with moms on Prozac were more irritable and colicky, symptoms that went away when the mother stopped taking it. If mom takes her dose of Prozac and discards the milk she pumps 7 to 10 hours later, her baby will receive 25% less drug in the milk. Another study showed that Zoloft (sertraline) is the only SSRI that shows a clear correlation between when mom takes the medication and when there is a peak in breast milk. The bottom line seems to be that if mom needs to be on medications, SSRIs are a reasonable choice while she is breastfeeding baby, with the possible exception of Prozac.

Women

Should women with premenstrual dysphoric disorder take antidepressants?

Q A

Perhaps. Because treatment for premenstrual dysphoric disorder (PMDD—discussed in Chapter 4) is much like that of major depression, antidepressants (especially SSRIs) are the mainstay of medical treatment.

Are antidepressants prescribed for women nearing menopause?

Q A

Often, yes. We know that Effexor (venlafaxine), Remeron (mirtazapine), and the SSRIs can help with hot flashes and treat depression, so these are often the ones chosen. The role of estrogen replacement continues to be hotly debated. Supplemental psychotherapy can help the woman deal with changes in role and identity at this time in her life. Studies are also looking at over-the-counter phytoestrogens (estrogen from a plant source; soy is probably the best known) and prescription sleep aids as alternatives.

The Elderly

Do antidepressants work differently in older adults?

Q A

Yes, they can. Antidepressants can be safely used in the elderly, but generally should be started at lower doses than in younger adults. Antidepressants may take longer to be effective in older people, so it can be helpful to add psychotherapy to "jump start" the recovery while the antidepressants are taking effect.

Electroconvulsive Therapy (ECT)

Electroconvulsive therapy (ECT) is a treatment that involves, under anesthesia, a brief electrical stimulation that causes an even briefer seizure in the brain.

Who is a good candidate for ECT?

Q A

ECT is a treatment usually reserved for the following:

- Depression is so severe that improvement must begin within days, not weeks
- Those who can't take oral medications or antidepressants
- Those who have failed trials of other medications and psychotherapies
- Depressions are marked by psychotic or manic symptoms
- Those for whom no other treatments have been effective

I thought "shock treatments" were a thing of the past. Not true?

Q A

Unfortunately, ECT has such a negative image from distorted views presented in movies and television that people are afraid of it, viewing it as an instrument of oppression or torture. Nothing could be further from the truth. ECT is a medical procedure usually performed in a hospital, either as an inpatient or even as an outpatient.

Not as Seen on TV
ECT has such a negative image from distorted views presented in movies and television that people are afraid of it, viewing it as an instrument of oppression or torture. Nothing could be further from the truth.

Q

What happens during ECT?

A

Patients are given basic blood work, an electrocardiogram to ensure heart health, and x-rays of the spine if there is a history of back problems. Patients and their families usually watch an educational video showing the treatment –a good time to ask any questions about the treatment or to discuss any concerns or fears before consenting. While under general anesthesia, the patient receives a muscle relaxant and stimulus pads are positioned on the scalp. The patient is asleep when a brief electrical stimulation causes an even briefer seizure in the brain. The patient sleeps through this and awakens after the procedure with few, if any, side effects. They don't feel anything during the course of the treatment and, because of the muscle relaxant, their bodies don't actually have a seizure.

Q

Are there any side effects to ECT?

A

At worst, people may have a mild headache and some memory loss for a brief period of time following treatment. Researchers have found no evidence that ECT directly damages the brain.

Q

What is the treatment regimen for ECT?

A

A usual course of ECT consists of about 10 to 12 treatments, given 2 to 3 times per week. Some patients require maintenance treatments of ECT to remain well, receiving them every 4 to 6 weeks, usually along with an antidepressant.

Vagal Nerve Stimulation (VNS)

Vagal nerve stimulation (VNS) is a new treatment for treatment-resistant depression that the FDA has recently approved.

Q

What is the vagus nerve?

A

The vagus, or "wandering" nerve, is one of the body's major nerves. It runs from the base of the brain down through the neck and chest to the stomach. It helps control the muscles that regulate heart rate and breathing, speaking, and digestive processes, and carries sensory information and impulses from the belly to the brain and back. This nerve also has fibers that effect the areas of the brain we believe are involved in regulating emotions and mood.

Q

Was VNS developed with treating depression in mind?

A

No. VNS was first used to treat uncontrolled epilepsy or seizures. It works like this: a device is connected to the vagus nerve in the neck. A small battery/pulse generator is implanted in the chest wall (like a heart pacemaker). When the device is turned on, the seizures are turned off! Investigators noted that some of these patients reported an improvement in depression, so doctors began to look at VNS as a treatment for difficult-to-treat depression.

The Seizure Connection
VNS was first used to treat uncontrolled epilepsy or seizures but doctors noticed that some of these patients reported an improvement in depression.

What happens during VNS?

Q A

The initial surgery to place the device is done in an outpatient surgical setting and takes an hour or two. Batteries in the device last 1 to 3 years, and changing the batteries and making adjustments to the device is easily done in the doctor's office.

Are there side effects to VNS?

Q A

Side effects are infrequent and minor, ranging from voice hoarseness, sore throat, problems swallowing, cough, and nausea, often improving with time.

Is there any evidence that VNS works?

Q A

The jury is still out on whether this treatment works, and many insurers won't pay for it (the procedure costs around $25,000). Patients must have failed at least four adequate trials of medication and/or ECT before receiving this treatment.

Repetitive Transcranial Magnetic Stimulation (rTMS)

Repetitive Transcranial Magnetic Stimulation (rTMS) is a treatment that uses specialized electromagnetic coils and electrical current to gently stimulate very specific parts of the brain without the need for anesthesia. It is thought to alter brain function in such a way as to alleviate depression.

What happens during rTMS?

Q A

A specialized electromagnetic coil is positioned over the patient's head and an electrical current is passed through it, creating a magnetic field. Each session lasts about a half hour, and are generally daily for 2 to 4 weeks.

Does rTMS have side effects?

Q A

Side effects are minimal with some patients complaining of scalp discomfort, dizziness, or headache, but generally not so much that they stop treatments. No memory problems have been reported.

No Need To "Go Under"
Think of rTMS as ECT-lite—a technique that gently stimulates the brain without the need for anesthesia.

Q

Is there any evidence that rTMS is effective?

A

We don't have enough hard evidence yet that this treatment is effective.

Light Therapy

Light therapy is the exposure to either natural or artificial light to regulate the pineal gland in the brain.

Q

How does light—or the absence of it—play a role in depression?

A

Who doesn't feel better, more energized, and happier on bright, sunny days? And some of us feel down, blue and sluggish on rainy, grey, overcast days. These are normal variations in our feelings that can occur in response to changes in light intensity and duration. Multiply these normal feelings over and over again and you can appreciate the overwhelming changes in mood that some people experience with changes in the amount of light they are exposed to. There are many theories about why humans can be so sensitive to these changes in light. The most important involves a small gland in our brain called the pineal gland. This gland secretes a substance called melatonin that may be a factor in stabilizing our moods and sleep, as well as affecting other functions–like appetite, sex, and energy.

The Sunshine Factor

Who doesn't feel better, more energized, and happier on bright, sunny days? And some of us feel down, blue and sluggish on rainy, grey, overcast days. These are normal variations in our feelings that can occur in response to changes in light intensity and duration.

Q

Everyone needs some light. How do we know how much is enough?

A

In some people there seems to be a "glitch" in the delicate balance of light and brain chemicals, and they go on to develop severe problems regulating their moods. Some people experience this seasonally, with an onset or worsening of their illness in the fall or winter, followed by remission in the spring or summer (oddly, some people experience this pattern in reverse!). If this occurs for 2 years in a row, it's known as *seasonal affective disorder (SAD)*. SAD can occur in about 1 to 5% of the population, with higher rates in more northern areas–those with less exposure to sunlight.

Q

What's the treatment for someone who needs more light?

A

SAD is treated as depression would be, but can be also treated with light therapy. For example, we know that regular exercise can help people feel better and relieve depression. If this exercise can be done outside during the day for at least 30 to 60 minutes, it may provide the extra sunlight a patient needs to ward off or relieve symptoms of depression. More than 70% of people who add this exercise/sunlight to their daily schedule report improvement in their depression, energy levels, and sex drive.

Q

What if no natural light is available?

A

For those who aren't able to get natural light, an alternative might be bright light therapy. One can buy light "boxes" that provide the appropriate high intensity light (10,000 lux) needed for a therapeutic effect. The most common way to get the light needed from the light box is to be exposed to it for 30 to 40 minutes daily. The light might be on while a person eats breakfast, reads the paper, exercises, or during another daily routine.

Q

Are there side effects to light therapy?

A

Most frequent side effects include headache, nausea, insomnia (if exposed to the light too close to bedtime), and eyestrain.

Is there any evidence that light therapy works?

Yes. By adding this light to their environment, up to 75% of people studied reported improvement in their mood and energy levels.

Psychotherapies

Psychotherapy, or talk therapy, can help people learn better ways of dealing with life's stresses and can modify the often distorted, negative thinking and behaviors that come with depression.

Banish Bad Thoughts

Psychotherapy can modify the often distorted, negative thinking and behaviors that come with depression.

Who is a good candidate for psychotherapy?

Almost anyone can benefit. Psychotherapy can be invaluable in sustaining a person while antidepressants are kicking in (which may take weeks to be fully effective). People often confuse therapy with what they have seen in the media: patients lying on couches, coming in every week for years to complain about their mothers!

Are therapists professionals?

Yes. Therapists can be many different medical professionals who all have advanced medical degrees or licenses (see Table 6-1).

Paging Dr. Freud

Psychotherapy is *not* patients lying on couches, coming in every week for years to complain about their mothers!

How long does a person have to be in psychotherapy?

In general, therapy tends to be brief and focused and last a few weeks or months, not years.

Is all psychotherapy the same?

No. There are hundreds of kinds of psychotherapies, just like there are hundreds of kinds of medications. Not all psychotherapies are well suited to treat depression, or are even effective. It's helpful to think about psychotherapy as another kind of medication, with specific types for specific illnesses.

Which psychotherapies are effective for depression?

We've found that two forms of therapy are just as effective as antidepressants in treating mild to moderate depressions (without psychosis or active suicidal thoughts):

- *Cognitive-behavioral therapy* and
- *Interpersonal therapy*

Q What is cognitive-behavioral therapy?

A *Cognitive-behavioral therapy,* at its most basic form, teaches that we feel what we think and act. Thus, negative thinking can lead to lowered self-esteem, which can lead to negative behaviors, social withdrawal and isolation, giving up or having no sense of purpose, and so on. The goal of the therapist who uses this technique is to interrupt this pattern by encouraging the patient to:

- Examine their negative thoughts and behaviors
- Change them to more positive ones
- Replace negative behaviors with more constructive ones
- Re-engage in pleasurable activities and
- Work toward achieving goals in healthier thinking and acting

In psychotherapy, small successes continue to build, providing positive reinforcement for the pattern to repeat.

Words from the Wise
Those who succeed in cognitive-behavioral therapy ultimately come to endorse what Winston Churchill, who suffered from severe depression, noted when he was in recovery: "I am an optimist. It does not seem too much use being anything else." Or, in the words of Abraham Lincoln: "Most people are about as happy as they make up their minds to be."

Q What is interpersonal therapy?

A *Interpersonal therapy* treats depression from a different perspective. It looks at the context of how relationships are affected in depression–how strained relationships and lack of support may lead to depression, and how ongoing depression damages relationships further, which leads to more depression, and so on. Interpersonal therapists attempt to correct distorted relationships. The goal is to reduce the symptoms of depression, and to help people develop new ways to relate to others, particularly where disputes or conflicts are involved.

Q Is psychotherapy alone effective?

A Although therapy along can be effective in treating mild to moderate depression, combining any therapy with an antidepressant medication helps patients get better quicker and maintain their wellness longer.

Complementary and Alternative Treatments

Sometimes people are ashamed to admit their depression, and will seek remedies that are out of the mainstream to ease their pain. Often, these people are wary of prescribed drugs or treatments, and will seek other therapies because they perceive them to be "safer" or "natural." What they do is to seek a *complementary* treatment (something *in addition to* medication and/or counseling) or *alternative* treatment (something *instead* of medication and/or counseling). These include:

- Herbs
- Supplements
- Acupuncture
- Exercise
- Meditation

We'll discuss each of these in detail.

People should discuss any remedies they have tried with their healthcare providers, as some of these agents—especially ones that are ingested—may not be safe if combined with other medications the patient may be taking.

Herbs

What's the history of using herbs to treat depression?

Plants, herbs, and flowers have a long history of being used for decreasing pain, curing illness, and restoring emotional balance.

What's the most common one used?

The most common herbal treatment for depression is St. John's Wort (*Hypericum perforatum*) shown in Figure 6-1. St. John's Wort is a low-growing bushy herb with yellow flowers, regarded as an invasive nuisance plant in many parts of the country. It blooms in June, the legendary birthday of St. John the Baptist (hence its name).

Is St. John's wort used only in this country?

No. St. John's Wort is actually a prescription antidepressant in Europe where it's commonly used to treat mild to moderate depression. It's even added to the feed of horses and cattle to make them more mellow and calm! It's thought to act much as the SSRIs—increasing the amount of serotonin in the brain. The use of St. John's Wort is centuries old and is increasing in popularity in the United States.

Is St. John's Wort effective for depression?

Well-designed scientific studies have demonstrated that it may be effective in relieving mild cases of depression as long as people aren't on any other medications with which this herb might interact. More studies are needed to show its true effectiveness.

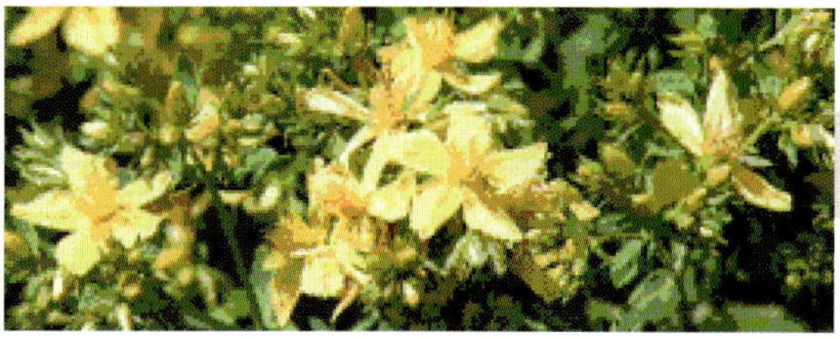

Figure 6-1. St. John's Wort.

Are there side effects to using St. John's Wort?

Headache, upset stomach, rash, and sensitivity to light are the most common side effects patients report. Otherwise it's relatively well tolerated. It takes just as long to act as traditional antidepressants–generally a few weeks.

I've heard there may be different levels of purity of St. John's Wort. Is this true?

It's absolutely true! Because St. John's Wort isn't regulated for purity and potency by the FDA, consumers might not be getting a pure, safe product. You could literally be buying grass clippings in a capsule!
Also, some patients assume that because an agent is "natural," it's safe and won't react badly to other medications they may be taking. Sadly, this isn't always the case. One study showed that some patients recovering from organ transplants who felt stressed or depressed and took St. John's Wort wound up rejecting their transplants because it lowered their anti-rejection drug levels.

Q

Does that mean I shouldn't take St. John's Wort if I'm taking other medications?

A

It depends on what other drugs you're taking. Other interactions we're aware of include the lowering of AIDs drug levels; a decrease in effectiveness of birth control pills; lowered levels of certain blood thinners (warfarin), heart rhythm drugs (digoxin), and asthma drugs (theophylline); and loss in power of some anti-cancer medications. This makes it even more important for people to tell their doctor that they're taking herbals like St. John's Wort.

Supplements

Supplements are a complementary treatment and refer to something that you ingest or take orally. The main ones that are used to treat depression are:

- SAM-e
- Omega-3 fatty acids and
- DHEA

SAM-e

Q

What does SAM-e do?

A

S-adenosyl-l-methionine (SAM-e) is an amino acid derivative that is a natural part of human brain cells. Taking SAM-e may increase levels of chemicals in the brain, such as serotonin and dopamine, which are important for maintaining emotional balance.

SAM-e

Taking SAM-e may increase levels of chemicals in the brain, such as serotonin and dopamine, which are important for maintaining emotional balance.

Q

Is SAM-e effective for treating depression?

A

Like St. John's Wort, SAM-e holds promise for the treatment of mild to moderate depression. It is well tolerated, with mild stomach upset and headache being the most common side effects. The most troublesome side effect, however, might be price, as it's costly and generally not covered by insurance. There are also questions about the appropriate dosage.

Q

Is there anyone who shouldn't take SAM-e?

A

People with bipolar depression shouldn't use SAM-e as there's a small risk of this agent causing a manic (or "up") episode.

Omega-3 fatty acids

Q

What do omega-3 fatty acids do?

A

Omega-3 fatty acids are necessary for the growth and nourishment of healthy brain cells and cell membranes.

Q

Are omega-3 fatty acids effective in treating depression?

A

Omega-3 fatty acids, also known as "fish oils," have become increasingly popular as either a sole treatment or an add-on treatment in depression. The interest in these compounds came about as scientists noted that, in countries where people ate more fish and foods higher in omega-3s (such as green leafy vegetables, walnuts, flaxseed, and soy), they seemed to have lower rates of depression. As American consumption of these foods lessened, our depression rates have soared. Anecdotal studies seem to indicate that omega-3s on their own may be helpful for mild depression. Side effects are low and these supplements aren't terribly expensive (see Table 6-3).

How does one take omega-3 fatty acids?

It's not yet clear what the lowest effective dose of these supplements is. Most doctors will counsel their patients to live more healthy lifestyles by getting better nutrition. They are comfortable counseling patients to use omega-3s as an add-on treatment to traditional medications and/or psychotherapy.

Go Fish

As American consumption of foods high in omega-3 fatty acids have lessened, our depression rates have soared.

Dehydroepiandrosterone (DHEA)

What does DHEA do?

DHEA (*Dehydroepiandrosterone)* is a steroid hormone secreted by the adrenal gland, and is one of the building blocks of estrogens and testosterone–the female and male hormones. DHEA has been marketed heavily to consumers as a means of "turning back the aging clock" to enhance physical strength, muscle mass, immunity, memory, sexual functioning, and mood.

Is DHEA effective in treating depression?

A recent study reported that DHEA was effective in half of their subjects in improving mild to moderate symptoms of depression, as well as sexual functioning. It also noted that there isn't much safety data concerning long-term use of this hormone. Short-term side effects include facial hair growth, deepened voice, spotty hair loss, and menstrual irregularities in women, and breast and prostate enlargement in men. Long-term side effects could include liver damage, increased heart disease in women, and stimulation of cancers sensitive to hormones (like prostate, breast, or endometrial cancer).

Is there anyone who shouldn't take DHEA?

Those younger than middle-aged or those with severe depression or who have histories of hormonally sensitive cancers or liver disease shouldn't take DHEA. Middle-aged patients who haven't responded to traditional means of treating depression and who don't have the risk factors listed above and have mild to moderate depression could consider DHEA treatment.

Acupuncture

What is acupuncture?

Acupuncture is a traditional Asian treatment that has been practiced for thousands of years. Needles are inserted at specific points in the body and either manually manipulated or electrically stimulated to correct imbalances of forces needed for optimal health (yin and yang forces), which also have an effect on the body's flow of energy (known as "Qi"). According to this Eastern school of thought, when imbalances in yin or yang or in Qi forces exist, disease can occur, including mental imbalance or depression. Western acupuncturists believe that acupuncture is effective because the manipulation of the needles affects the levels of brain chemicals important to emotional balance—norepinephrine and serotonin.

The Skinny on Needles

Two schools of thought exist on why acupuncture works:

- In the Eastern school of thought, when imbalances in yin or yang or in Qi forces exist, disease can occur, including mental imbalance or depression.
- In the Western school of thought, acupuncture needles affect the levels of the brain chemicals norepinephrine and serotonin.

Q

Is there anyone who shouldn't have acupuncture?

A

Acupuncture is relatively safe, with few side effects and no drug-drug interactions. The technique has been used on millions of Americans, usually for the relief of pain.

Q

Is acupuncture effective for treating depression?

A

We don't have a lot of evidence to prove that it is, and few insurers will cover it for depression. More rigorous studies are needed.

Q

Exercise

How can exercise work in treating depression?

A

Exercise can help lift depression because it can:

- Increase the natural brain chemicals known as endorphins, which act as natural antidepressants
- Reduce levels of harmful stress hormones
- Enhance overall physical health and increase social interaction
- Distract patients from their worries and depressive thoughts
- Enhance a person's sense of self-worth and take away some of the poor self-esteem found in depression

Q

Is exercise effective in treating depression?

A

The answer appears to be a qualified yes (Table 6-5). Good, well-controlled studies are hard to find, but the few available seem to suggest that moderate exercise can reduce the symptoms of depression, especially if people can stick with it for at least 13 weeks. Medications seemed to produce a quicker response, but people who also exercised seemed to keep their symptoms in remission longer. People who exercise on their own find that it is cheap, readily available, and (if done correctly) relatively safe. Cost will increase if you use trainers, fitness clubs, or exercise equipment. The limiting factor is a person's "get up and go," since depression is an illness marked by both fatigue and lack of motivation.

Q

How would one use exercise to treat depression?

A

When a doctor starts a medication, he or she may "start low and go slow" to avoid side effects. We can approach a "prescription" for exercise the same way. We don't tell patients to go out and run a mile every other day. We might counsel them to walk 5 minutes on their treadmill twice a week, and write it down. The next week try it three times a week, and write it down. The next time, make it 10 minutes three times a week, again, writing it down. Small successes will lead to larger ones. Take the final goal and break it down into small steps. It's also ok to miss a day. Remember that tomorrow is another day. Three steps forward, one back. Even that progress means your motion is going forward!

Table 6-5: Benefits of Exercise

- Free
- Portable
- Under the patient's control
- Generally free of side effects
- Possible weight loss
- Better heart health
- An improved sense of overall well-being
- Can be tailored to individual needs
- Can be "mixed up" to help maintain interest
- Can relieve feelings of being withdrawn or isolated by finding a buddy or a group to exercise with

Q

Who is a good candidate to use exercise for depression?

A

If a person has a mild depression, still has "get up and go," would rather not take a medication, and has no severe life stressors that appear to have triggered the depression, then exercise alone might be an acceptable first-line treatment. Small, achievable goals—start low, go slow—must be the rule.

Q

Is there anyone who shouldn't exercise as part of their depression treatment?

A

If a person is already demoralized and without energy or has severe symptoms, an exercise program as the sole treatment may be doomed to fail. With this type of person, exercise can be introduced later in the treatment plan as part of a balanced plan to get the person all the way well, both physically and mentally.

Meditation

Q

What is meditation?

A

Meditation has a variety of meanings depending upon whom you ask. For some, it's thoughtful contemplation. For others, it's a more formal inner discipline of focusing one's conscious awareness to lead to a spiritually enlightened state.

Q

Who are good candidates to use meditation to treat depression?

A

Those with mild depression are the ones most likely to try meditation and relaxation practices.

Q

Is meditation effective in treating depression?

A

Despite its popularity, there isn't much published data showing the effectiveness of meditation as a treatment for depression. Some mental health workers worry that encouraging severely depressed patients to meditate could be counterproductive, as these people find it nearly impossible to concentrate and focus. Failure to be successful at meditation could lead to further demoralization or depression. Some studies suggest, however, that if people on the path to wellness are taught how to meditate they might be able to stay well longer by being able to process their negative thoughts and feelings more constructively.

CHAPTER SEVEN

Can Depression Be Cured?

Treatments continue to improve all the time, and 70 to 90% of depressed patients, if treated correctly, will get well, and can get *all the way well.*

Q

If I feel well, can't I stop whatever medicine I'm taking?

A

Not right away. When you feel like you've gotten all the way well and continue to feel this way, you should continue to take the antidepressant for at least 6 to 12 months before making any decision about stopping. At that point, if you have risk factors for depression (covered in Chapter 3), you should realize that stopping treatment could cause the depression to come back. The dose of medication that got you well will keep you well.

Q

What will happen if I do stop taking medication?

A

If you do wean yourself off the medication you are taking (stopping gradually and *never* stopping taking medication abruptly), you may not respond as well to the same treatment if the depression returns.

Antidepressants: Don't Stop Too Soon
Stay on your medical treatment for 6 to 12 months: if you have risk factors for depression, stopping treatment can cause depression to come back.

Q

How can I stay well and avoid depression?

A

If you successfully participated in psychotherapy to relieve your depression, addressing some of the factors that may have led to or maintained your depression will likely lessen the chance that it will come back. You can discuss this more with your mental health care provider. Table 7-1 provides additional tips for keeping depression away.

Table 7-1: Keeping Depression Away: What You Can Do

- Stay on treatment regimen 6 to 12 months before considering stopping
- Realize that stopping treatment can cause the depression to return
- Understand that if you stop your medication, you may not respond as well with the same regimen if the depression returns
- If in therapy, address the factors that may have led to the depression
- Discussion treatment decisions carefully with your health care professional

Q

Does depression ever really go away completely?

A

For most people, depression is more chronic than not. It's more like arthritis than appendicitis. When someone is in treatment for depression, the goal of the treatment needs to be to get *all the way well*, as smoldering symptoms of low-level depression greatly increase the risk of relapse. The good news is that depression can often be overcome.

CHAPTER EIGHT

Can Depression Be Fatal?

Depression is an illness—and it can be fatal. Somewhere between 10 to 15% percent of depressed patients will die by their own hand each year, accounting for at least 30,000 victims a year.

The Bottom Line
Depression can be fatal. Suicide claims 30,000 lives a year—10 to 15% of depressed patients.

Where does suicide rank in overall fatalities in the United States?

Q

A

There are actually more suicides than homicides committed yearly in the United States. This number may be greatly underestimated due to the stigma of suicide and issues regarding loss of insurance benefits if reported.

Is there any segment of the population that suicide affects most?

Q

A

Men commit suicide more often than women, although women make more suicide attempts.

Does everyone who is depressed contemplate suicide?

Q

A

No, not everyone who is depressed contemplates suicide. On the other hand, no one who suffers from depression is immune from this most dangerous and possibly lethal symptom.

Can you predict someone's suicide?

Q

A

It's so hard to predict an event that only affects a small part of the population. And in truth, if someone is bent on killing themselves, they most likely won't reveal it to family, friends, or their health care providers. If someone you care about is depressed, you must look for clues in their history and behavior. There are some "red flags" (Table 8-1) that can alert you to the possibility that suicidal thinking or behavior could exist.

Table 8-1: "Red Flags" That Can Indicate Suicide

- Severe depression or anxiety
- Previous history of suicidal thinking or a suicide attempt
- Family history of suicide
- Older age
- Male gender
- Ongoing alcohol or drug abuse
- Recent loss (e.g., partner, job)
- Recent diagnosis of terminal or disabling disease
- Lack of social support
- Clear plan for suicide with means of carrying it out

Q If I think someone is contemplating suicide what should I do?

A If you're worried about this possibility in someone, *go ahead and ask them,* openly and kindly. Asking about it doesn't permit them to do it or encourage them to go forward. It may open up a dialogue that lets you get the person to emergency help.

Q I've contemplated suicide. Sometimes it seems like the only way out.

A You must seek help, and realize that it's the depression that makes things seem so bleak. *There is help and comfort available.* The pain and suffering that suicide will leave behind in your family and friends is intolerable.

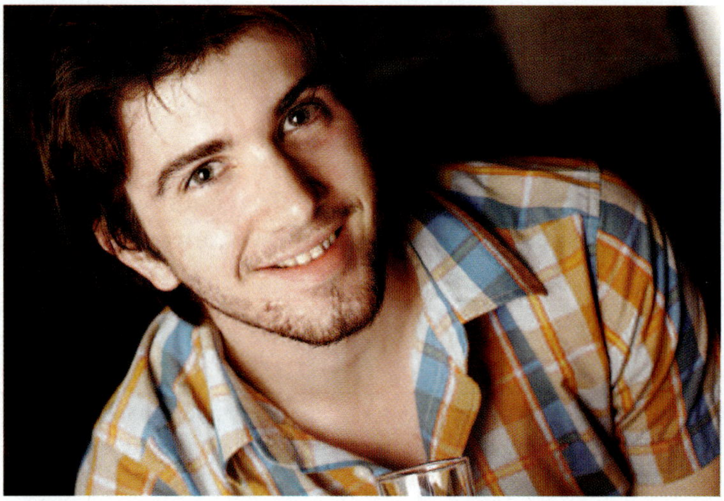

all the way well

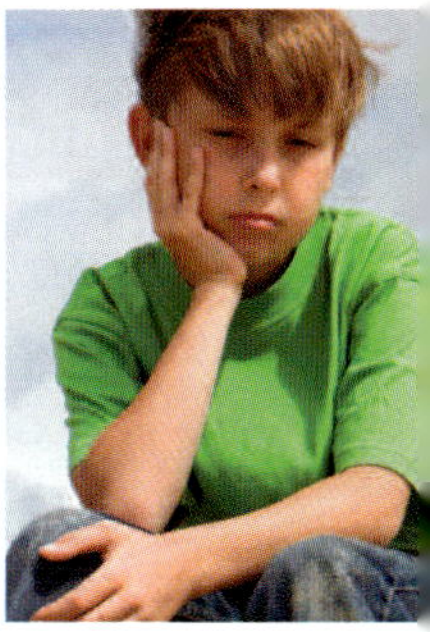

CHAPTER NINE

I'm Depressed – What Should I Know?

Depression is sneaky and evil. It causes you to look at the world in a distorted way. It makes you feel like there's no hope, that it's not worth going on, or that you should give up. Chapter 11, *Where Can I Find Help?*, will give you some resources for information that can help you.

Depression Is Sneaky and Evil
Depression causes you to look at the world in a distorted way, makes you feel like there's no hope, that it's not worth going on, and that you should give up.

Sometimes I feel like the depression is my fault. Could it be? Q

A No. Depression is an illness and you didn't choose to be depressed—and you aren't weak or crazy. You must understand that this is the depression speaking.

Can treatment really help me? Q

A If you begin a treatment program, one thing that will begin to happen is your negative thinking will fade as any medical treatments begin to work, especially if you are involved with psychotherapy, too. There really is hope, it is worth going on, and you should never, ever give up! It takes time for the treatments to take effect, but they will work. *You can get better.* Table 9-1 offers some key things you need to know about your depression.

Do other people with depression feel the same as me? Q

A Probably not exactly the same. Depression is *not* the same for everyone. There are many different causes and treatments. That's why it's so important to work with your doctors to come up with an individualized, balanced plan to guide you in getting back to *all the way* well.

I just wish my depression could lift now. How long do I have to wait for relief? Q

A Recovery from depression is a series of small steps. Start slowly to re-enter yourself into the pattern of your life. Keep the lines of communication open with friends and family. Each small success in achieving a goal will build upon itself. Even if you take a few steps forward and have a step back, you are still going forward. Easy does it: do what you can, when you can.

Table 9-1: Your Depression: Key Points on the Road to Recovery

- Acknowledge that depression is an illness—you didn't choose to be here
- Expect your negative thinking to begin to fade as your treatment begins to work
- Establish an individual plan to steer you through—no one's depression is the same as yours
- Know that recovery comes in small steps
- Take any prescribed medications every day—don't take more and don't take less
- Call your doctor with any questions at all
- Rely on family, friends, support groups—pain shared is pain made more bearable
- Don't make any decisions while depressed—postpone them until you have a more balanced perspective
- Get moving! Exercise generally helps
- Believe that you will get well

Q

Do I really have to make my medications every day for them to work?

A

Take your prescribed medications every day. If side effects are troublesome, call your doctor. There might be very simple things that can be done to help you feel better until your body gets used to the medicine. Most importantly, don't take more in the hope that you will get better faster, and don't stop any medication abruptly without telling your doctor. Don't drink alcohol or use it to get to sleep; if you are having sleep problems tell your doctor. Call your doctor with *any* questions at all. Your treatment team is there to help!

Your medications:

- Take them every day
- Don't take more: you won't get better faster
- Don't stop abruptly: if any changes need to be made, tell your doctor

Q

I hate to burden my friends and family with my depression. Should I?

A

Don't feel badly for leaning on your family and friends. You would do the same for them if the tables were turned. Participate in support groups or group therapy— pain shared is pain made more bearable. Those who have been on the path to wellness longer than you can have valuable insights to share.

Q

More often than not, I feel so lethargic, like I just don't want to move. How do I overcome this?

A

If you are at all able, try to exercise a little. Get moving. Go out. Get to the mall, a movie, a church group. Reach out to other people; more often than not they will reach back.

Worth the Wait

You can slowly, but surely, feel better. Recovery takes time.

Q

I feel so scattered sometimes or tempted to do things I think will make the depression better.

A

While you are depressed isn't the time to make important decisions, especially important life decisions like changing jobs or getting married or divorced. Postpone them until you feel better and have a more balanced perspective on life. Wait until you are feeling better and your thinking becomes clearer. Set realistic goals.

CHAPTER TEN

I Know Someone Who is Depressed: What Should I Know

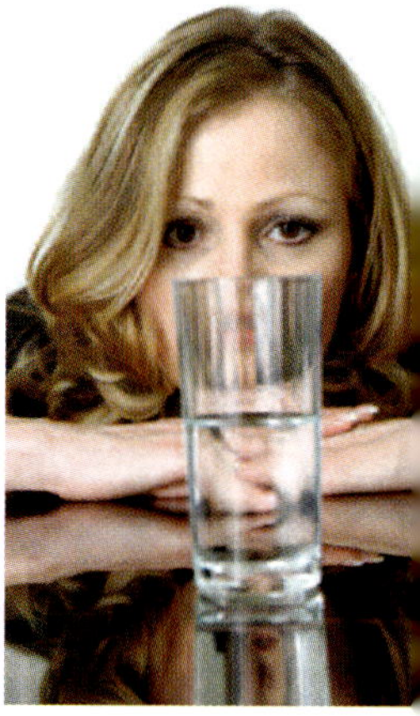

Family and friends are a tremendous source of support for their loved ones with depression. The illness, by its very nature, causes its victims to withdraw and isolate. Those of us who care need to continuously bring our loved ones out of the darkness and back into the light. Chapter 11, *Where Can I Find Help?*, will give you some resources for information that can help you.

Q
A

What's the most important thing I can do for someone who I suspect is depressed?

The most critical thing you can do is to steer them to a medical professional to get the correct diagnosis and treatment. You can help reduce the stigma of depression by acknowledging that depression, like high blood pressure or cancer, is a medical illness that can get better with medical treatment. Table 10-1 also provides some suggestions for handling someone else's depression.

Acknowledge that Depression Is an Illness
You can help reduce the stigma of depression by acknowledging that depression, like high blood pressure or cancer, is a medical illness that can get better with medical treatment.

Table 10-1: When You Know Someone Who is Depressed

What you can do for *them*	What you can do for *you*
• Steer them toward professional help • Consider making initial and follow-up appointments for them, then going for support and back-up • Once in treatment, encourage them to stay there • Help them make healthy choices: no alcohol, healthier eating, exercise	• Acknowledge that depression is an illness, not a choice • Be patient; recovery is a slow process • Try not to feel hurt or rejected; their depression isn't about *you*

Q Can my loved one get better without treatment?

A If he or she is truly depressed, probably not. It's not likely that they can snap out of depression on their own—that would be like asking or expecting someone with cancer or diabetes to snap out of their illness without treatment! Once a diagnosis is made and treatment begins, you can and should do the following:

- Encourage them to *stay* in treatment, as recovery is a slow process.
- If you have to, make the initial and follow-up appointments and go with them for support and back-up.
- Encourage them to take their medication, even if it seems to take forever to take effect.
- Steer them away from alcohol and help them make healthy choices that will speed their recovery: healthier eating, mild exercise, and gratifying activities.

Q My friend seems to be improving, but so slowly.

A You need to realize that small baby steps are important at first, then bigger ones as the person begins to emerge from the dark cocoon of depression. Don't settle for better. Encourage them to get all the way to *best.*

Q I wish I could get inside my depressed friend's mind. What could she be thinking that is so bleak?

A It's important to realize that people with depression often feel hopeless, helpless, and worthless. This is part of their illness and not an accurate reflection of the way things really are. It's difficult (if not impossible) to know how terrible depression feels and how it distorts reasonable thinking, unless you have been there yourself. Family and friends can be a vital resource in continually reflecting back that things aren't so bleak, that the illness is causing them to feel so pessimistic, and that these feelings will fade as their treatment progresses.

Q Is there anything I shouldn't say?

A Try not to be glib with comments like "just get over it" or "I know just how you feel." Remind them of their strengths and successes.

Q Should I take all suicide threats seriously or trust my instincts in this matter?

A Don't minimize any comments about suicide or self-harm. Call the treating doctor or therapist immediately. If harm seems imminent, call 911. Don't worry about causing a fuss or having your loved one be angry with you later. You could be saving a life. If your loved one's life is in danger and they won't accept the recommendation to come in to the hospital, you may have the ability to sign them in for care involuntarily. Don't hesitate to do this, even if you fear that they will be angry with you. You could be saving their life (fig 10-1).

Q I miss the friend I used to know. Of course, I'm sorry for him, but I feel bad, too.

A Try to avoid feeling hurt or rejected. Your relationship with your loved one or friend will most certainly be tested. Remember, this illness isn't your fault. And take care of yourself and your own needs during this time—you won't be any use to your loved one if you become ill yourself.

CHAPTER ELEVEN

Where Can I Find Help?

If you are depressed, or if there is someone in your life that you care about who is depressed, the very *best* place to start is with a family doctor who can begin the diagnostic and treatment process. If there is an emergency situation, call or go to the nearest hospital emergency room.

However, other resources are widely available, especially:

- **Local services.** Check the phone book and look in the governmental resource pages (usually blue pages) under topics such as "Mental health," "Crisis intervention," "Counselors," and "Suicide hot line."
- **The Internet.** The Internet is a broad tool that is widely available and accessible to just about everyone these days. Some sites are quite good, but others can be inaccurate.

The following sites are high-quality, reliable places to begin on the journey to finding out more about depression. Knowledge is power and power is what you need to combat this potentially deadly illness. Phone numbers and addresses are provided where available.

General Information

National organizations

National Institutes of Health
www.nlm.nih.gov/medlineplus/depression.html
Lists resources and links concerning mental illness and depression, from diagnosis to comprehensive treatments to special populations
www.nimh.nih.gov (Click on the "Health information tab" then either "Bipolar disorder" or "Depression")
Offers information and reputable links
Available in Spanish
Also available at 1-800-421-4211 or via mail at NIMH, Information Resources and Inquiries Branch, 6001 Executive Boulevard, Room 8184 MSC 9663, Bethesda, MD 20892-9663

National Mental Health Information Center
www.mentalhealth.samhsa.gov
Lists hotline numbers
Links to other reputable resources

National Mental Health Association
www.nmha.org
Addresses all aspects of mental health and illness
Also available at 1-800-969-NMHA (6642) or via mail at 2001 North Beauregard Street 12th floor, Alexandria, VA 22311

www.depression-screening.org
Offers a brief screening test to see if a person might be depressed
Information and links about depression and its treatment
Free written information on many mental health topics
Lists local organizations and support groups
Also available at 1-800-969-6642

American Psychiatric Association
www.psych.org (Click on "Public Information")
Provides information on all aspects of depression and other mental illnesses
Provides information on finding a psychiatrist
Also available at 1-888-357-7924 and via mail at 1000 Wilson Boulevard Suite 1825, Arlington, VA 22209
www.healthyminds.org
A clearinghouse of information about mental illnesses and depression
Provides many helpful links

American Psychological Association
http://helping.apa.org
Provides broad educational resources on depression and other mental illnesses
Provides information on finding a psychologist
Also available at 1-800-964-2000

Depression and Bipolar Support Alliance
www.dbsalliance.org
Offers information on mood disorders, support groups and chapter locations
Also available at 1-800-826-3632 or via mail at 730 North Franklin Street, Suite 501, Chicago, IL 60610-7224

National Alliance on Mental Illness
www.nami.org
Links to resources and support groups
Gives the perspective of those who have lived with and survived depression
Also available at 1-800-950-NAMI (6264) or via mail at Colonial Place Three, 2107 Wilson Boulevard, Suite 300, Arlington, VA 22201-3042

International Foundation for Research and Education on Depression
www.ifred.org
Supports research into causes and cures
Provides support for those who suffer from depression and those who care for them
Also available at 1-800-789-2647

Geisinger Health System
www.geisinger.org (Click on "Health and wellness," then "Mental health")
Provides information on depression and treatments

Mayo Clinic
www.mayoclinic.com
Provides information on depression and treatment resources

Other sites

www.freedomfromfear.com
National non-profit mental health advocacy association
Provides referral sources

www.depressioncenter.net
Screening tools, mood journals, online support groups, and general information about depression for patients and their families
Links to other online resources

www.familyaware.org
Dedicated to helping the families of those suffering from depression learn about the condition
Information on finding resources for treatment and support

www.mentalhealthchannel.net
Provides comprehensive information about depression and other mental and physical disorders
Lists treatment and support resources

Medications

National Institutes of Health
www.nlm.nih.gov/medlineplus
Information about prescription and nonprescription medications

Physician's Desk Reference
www.gettingwell.com
Sponsored by the writers of the Physician's Desk Reference (PDR)
Contains the same information available to doctors translated into plain English for patients

Complementary and alternative treatments

National Center for Complementary and Alternative Medicine
http://nccam.nih.gov
Government clearinghouse on complementary and alternative medical treatments
Links to other reliable resources

American Heart Association
www.justmove.org
Geared to helping people establish a reasonable, healthy exercise program

Suicide prevention

www.hopeline.com
Provides resources and referral lines for those struggling for suicidal thoughts and feelings and the people who care for them
Also available at 1-800-SUICIDE (1-800-784-2433)

Women

Massachusetts General Hospital
www.womensmentalhealth.org
Spotlights mental health disorders associated with reproductive function

University of Michigan Health System
www.med.umich.edu/womensguide
A woman's guide to understanding depression

Men

National Institutes of Health
http://menanddepression.nimh.nih.gov
Focuses on the unique characteristics and needs of men with depression
Part of the "Real Men, Real Depression" campaign

Children and adolescents

American Academy of Child and Adolescent Psychiatry
www.aacap.org
Information on child and adolescent mood disorders
Help in finding a child and adolescent psychiatrist

The elderly

American Association for Geriatric Psychiatry
www.aagpgpa.org
Offers news, facts, tools, and expert information for adults coping with mental health issues and aging and their caregivers

American Association of Retired Persons
www.aarp.org (Click on "Health" then "AARP Health Guide" then "Depression")
Information on late-life depression and help for patients and caregivers
Also available at 1-800-424-3410 or via mail at 601 E Street, NW, Washington, DC 20049

Alcoholic or addicted patients

Alcoholics Anonymous
www.aa.org
Dedicated to helping people become clean and sober
Also available at 1-212-870-3400

Al-Anon
www.al-anon.alateen.org
Offers help and resources to families and teens affected by alcoholism in those they love
Also available at 1-888-425-2666

National Council on Alcoholism and Drug Dependence, Inc.
www.ncadd.org
Offers educational materials and information on alcoholism
Provides information on local treatment resources
Also available at 1-800-NCA-CALL (1-800-622-2255)

Glossary

Acupuncture is a traditional Asiatic treatment involving inserting needles at specific points in the body. The needles are manipulated manually or stimulated electrically to correct imbalances of forces needed for optimal health, including mental health.

Alternative medicine describes some something you can do or take for an illness such as depression that is *instead* of medication and/or counseling.

Auditory hallucinations are "voices" inside a person that only that person can "hear."

Can occur in the severely depressed.

Bipolar disorder is a depressive disorder with two "poles," one high and one low, which cycle back and forth.

Black box warning is a warning on prescription drug labeling that describes the increased risk of suicide in pediatric patients and emphasizes the need for closely monitoring patients started on these medications.

Cognitive-behavioral therapy is a branch of psychotherapy that teaches that we feel what we think and act.

Clinical depression is depression whose symptoms severely interfere with a person's ability to live well and function. Also known as unipolar or major depression.

Complementary medicine describes something you can do or take for an illness such as depression that is *in addition to* medication and/or counseling.

Delusions are false but unshakeable beliefs that mirror a depressed individual's poor self-esteem and hopelessness.

Depression is a persistent feeling of sadness that doesn't go away. It is characterized by a recognized set of symptoms. See also the definitions of major depression, minor depression, unipolar depression, bipolar disorder, and clinical depression.

DHEA (Dehydroepiandrosterone) is a steroid hormone secreted by the adrenal gland. It has been recognized to improve mild to moderate depression when taken as a dietary supplement.

Diagnostic and Statistical Manual, version 4 (DSM-4) is the standard mental health diagnosis reference book. This manual contains all the signs and symptoms of the major mental disorders, including depression.

Dysthymia is characterized by the same recognized symptoms as major depression that last at least two years at a low level, but usually not enough to disable a person. Also known as minor depression.

Electroconvulsive therapy (ECT) is a treatment that involves, under anesthesia, a brief electrical stimulation that causes an even briefer seizure in the brain.

Exercise can be used to alleviate mild to moderate symptoms of depression by increasing a group of natural brain chemicals known as endorphins, which act as natural antidepressants. It may also reduce levels of harmful stress hormones.

Interpersonal therapy is a branch of psychotherapy that looks at the context of how relationships are affected in depression—how strained relationships and lack of support can lead to depression and how ongoing depression damages relationships further.

Light therapy is the exposure to either natural or artificial light to regulate the pineal gland in the brain. The pineal gland secretes melatonin, which may be a factor in stabilizing moods.

Major depression is depression whose symptoms severely interfere with a person's ability to live well and function. Also known as unipolar or clinical depression.

Mania refers to one of the "poles" of bipolar disorder and is characterized by excess energy, pressured speech, and racing thoughts.

Meditation is thoughtful contemplation or a more formal inner discipline of focusing one's conscious awareness to lead to a spiritually enlightened state. Meditation is performed in the hopes of alleviating mild depression.

Minor depression is characterized by the same recognized symptoms as major depression that last at least two years at a low level, but usually not enough to disable a person. Also known as dysthymia.

Monoamine oxidase inhibitors (MAOIs) are an older class of medications that affect the enzymes that break down the brain chemicals norepinephrine and serotonin, making more of them available to the brain...

Off-label describes the way medications are appropriately used by doctors even though the U.S. Food and Drug Administration hasn't specifically approved them for a particular use.

Omega-3 fatty acids are present in fish and certain other foods. Scientists noted that there were lower rates of depression in countries where people ingested more omega-3 fatty acids.

Post-partum depression is depression following childbirth and is brought on by physical and hormonal changes. It is a major depressive episode that requires aggressive treatment and care. Post-partum depression isn't the syndrome known as "baby blues," which is quite common and involves passing, not persistent, feelings of sadness, fatigue, and fear.

Premenstrual dysphoric disorder (PMDD) is a mood disorder related to the timing of a woman's menstrual cycle. More than just "premenstrual syndrome, or PMS," it is more like a major depressive disorder with a formally recognized set of symptoms.

Psychosis describes a state of severely disorganized thinking, with speech and behavior that is irrational and incoherent. These individuals often have both auditory hallucinations and delusions.

Psychotherapy is essentially "talk" therapy performed by professionals. It's used to help people learn better ways of dealing with life's stresses and can often modify the distorted, negative thinking and behaviors that accompany depression.

Repetitive Transcranial Magnetic Stimulation (rTMS) is a treatment that uses specialized electromagnetic coils and electrical current to gently stimulate very specific parts of the brain without the need for anesthesia. It is thought to alter brain function in such a way as to alleviate depression.

Seasonal affective disorder (SAD) is a seasonal pattern of mood disturbance where there is either an onset or worsening of symptoms of depression in the fall or winter, followed by remission in the spring or summer. This needs to occur for 2 seasons in a row to be considered SAD.

SAM-e (S-adenosyl-l-methionine) is an amino acid derivative that is a natural part of human brain cells. Taking SAM-e may increase levels of the brain chemicals serotonin and dopamine, which are important for maintaining emotional balance.

Selective serotonin re-uptake inhibitors (SSRIs) are a class of medications that work by increasing the level of the brain chemical serotonin, which is important in regulating emotions and mood level.

St. John's wort is an herb that can be used to treat mild to moderate depression.

Tricyclic antidepressants (TCAs) are the oldest class of antidepressants. They work by affecting the brain chemicals norepinephrine and serotonin in varying amounts.

Unipolar depression is depression whose symptoms severely interfere with a person's ability to live well and function. Also known as major or clinical depression.

Vagal Nerve Stimulation (VNS) is a treatment that involves a small battery/pulse generator implanted in the chest wall that is connected to the vagus nerve. Among many other things, the vagus nerve has fibers that affect the areas of the brain we believe are involved in regulating emotions and mood.

all the way well